UNDERSTANDING
EPM

YOUR **GUIDE** TO HORSE HEALTH CARE AND MANAGEMENT

Copyright © 1997 The Blood-Horse, Inc.
All Rights reserved. No part of this book may be reproduced in any form by any means, including photocopying, audio recording, or any information storage or retrieval system, without the permission in writing from the copyright holder. Inquiries should be addressed to Publisher, The Blood-Horse, Inc., Box 4038, Lexington, KY 40544-4038.

ISBN 0-939049-93-7

Printed in the United States of America

First Edition: December 1997

1 2 3 4 5 6 7 8 9 10

UNDERSTANDING
EPM
Equine Protozoal Myeloencephalitis

YOUR **GUIDE** TO HORSE HEALTH CARE AND MANAGEMENT

By David E. Granstrom DVM, PhD

The Blood-Horse, Inc. Lexington, KY

Other titles offered by
The Horse **Health Care Library**

Understanding Equine Lameness

Understanding Equine First Aid

Understanding The Equine Foot

Understanding Equine Nutrition

Understanding Laminitis

Contents

Foreword by Stephen M. Reed,
  DVM, Diplomate ACVIM 6

Introduction 8
  History of the disease 11

Chapter 1 16
  What causes EPM?

Chapter 2 34
  What are the clinical signs of EPM?

Chapter 3 44
  How Is EPM diagnosed?
  Case Review I 70
  Case Review II 72
  Neurological Exam 74

Chapter 4 76
  How is EPM treated?

Chapter 5 84
  How Can EPM be prevented?

  Frequently Asked Questions 88
  Glossary of Terms 92
  Index 96
  Recommended Readings 98
  Photo Credits 102
  About The Author 103

FOREWORD

Although equine protozoal myeloencephalitis (EPM) has been recognized by its clinical symptoms since the mid-1960s, it has only recently been recognized as the most significant and important cause of spinal ataxia in horses in North America. We do not fully understand why it appears to have been only recently that the disease has become such a significant problem. The discovery of the causative protozoan parasite and the development of a diagnostic test, which is useful to distinguish this disease from other causes of spinal ataxia, have been instrumental in furthering our understanding within recent years.

The identification of *Sarcocystis neurona* as the causative organism and recognition that this organism is most likely *Sarcocystis falcatula* have provided us with a great deal of knowledge about the definitive host, parasite life cycle, and intermediate host(s) of this organism. This knowledge has helped us to begin to understand many of the risk factors which explain why so many horses are exposed to this disease. These discoveries also have helped us to understand why so many horses, horse owners, and veterinarians are so alarmed by EPM and the clinical problems associated with this disease.

Many researchers are to be complimented for their important scientific and clinical studies on this disease. However, the work of Dr. David Granstrom, along with his leadership and mentorship of Dr. Clara Fenger, was instrumental. Dr. Granstrom took his initial lead from Dr. J. P. Dubey, a renowned protozoologist, and later forged his own paths to develop a useful diagnostic test and study the biology of this organism. Their work has been complemented by Drs. John Dame and Rob McKay in Florida, Drs. Pat Conrad and Antoinette Marsh in California, and Drs. William Saville, Paul Morley, and me in Ohio.

Through the work of these investigators, we are well on the way to diagnosis, treatment, and control of this devastating disease of the horse and may soon lessen the medical and financial impact which this disease presents for the horse industry and the veterinary profession. I have personally examined more than 1,000 horses suffering from this difficult and often debilitating disease. I commend Dr. Granstrom for his diligence and thank him for his work and for the knowledge he is providing through this important text.

Stephen M. Reed, DVM, Diplomate ACVIM
Professor and Chief of Equine Medicine and Surgery
Department of Veterinary Clinical Sciences
The Ohio State University

INTRODUCTION

Equine protozoal myeloencephalitis (EPM) is the most commonly diagnosed equine neurologic disease in North America. Unfortunately, it presents a number of perplexing problems for owners and veterinarians that also make it one of the most difficult diseases to understand. Although a great deal has been learned about EPM since it first was described in the early 1960s, we are still far from fully understanding it today. Isolation of *Sarcocystis neurona*, the parasite that causes EPM, and the subsequent development of a laboratory diagnostic test in 1991 touched off an explosion of interest in EPM. It soon was learned that EPM was the real culprit in many clinical problems that had been incorrectly diagnosed or had not been diagnosed at all. The EPM test was used to determine exposure rates that approached 50% among the general horse population in several states. Seemingly overnight, EPM became the diagnosis *du jour*.

EPM has been found only in horses that originated in the Western Hemisphere. Although cases have been reported from Europe, Australia, and Africa, the affected horses were imported from the West. The first cases of EPM recognized in North America were from the Northeast. The disease now is recognized throughout the United States and southern Canada, as well as Central and South America. It is uncommon in the arid western United States, but the transient nature of the horse population has resulted in many confirmed cases, even from the desert Southwest. EPM affects all breeds at almost any age, but it seems concentrated in Thoroughbreds and Standardbreds under four years of age.

One of the foremost problems associated with EPM simply has been arriving at an accurate diagnosis. Clinical signs of the disease are so varied that it easily can be confused with almost

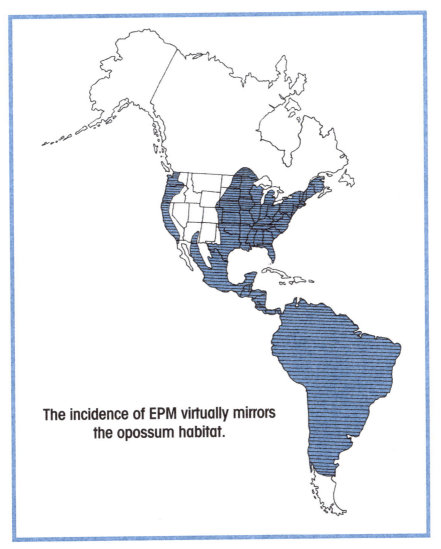

The incidence of EPM virtually mirrors the opossum habitat.

Introduction

any equine neurologic disease, and many non-neurologic diseases as well. Horses might be affected so mildly that it is difficult to detect a problem, or so severely that they are unable to stand. The disease can strike rapidly or insidiously, but most commonly produces gradually progressive incoordination and/or weakness of one or both rear limbs. Laboratory diagnosis has been a tremendous help, although some confusion and controversy regarding appropriate interpretation of test results have persisted.

> **AT A GLANCE**
>
> - Veterinary pathologists in the 1960s first recognized the disease that would become known as EPM.
>
> - In 1976, Dr. J. P. Dubey, then at The Ohio State University, identified the parasite as a species of *Sarcosystis*.
>
> - During the late 1970s, researchers described many of the clinical signs of EPM to help distinguish it from other equine neurologic diseases; during this time, blood tests were developed to detect antibodies to *Sarcocystis*.
>
> - The parasite was cultured by Dr. Dubey at the USDA-ARS, and a parasite-specific EPM diagnostic test was developed at the University of Kentucky in 1991.
>
> - A DNA test for *S. neurona* was developed in 1994.

Another problem area has involved effective treatment. Although some diversity of opinion still exists, it has taken years for a relatively standard treatment regimen to evolve. Some horses have made dramatic recoveries following treatment, while others have completely failed to respond. Nonetheless, the majority (55-65%) of horses responds favorably to treatment. Unfortunately only a fairly small percentage, possibly as high as 10%, recovers completely. It is most common for horses to make significant improvement over two to four months, then gradually plateau with some slight residual weakness or incoordination.

The need for persistent treatment of some horses to avoid relapse following complete or partial recovery has been another difficult problem to resolve. It is possible that the dosage recommendations used in the current standard treatment regimen are still too low. A group of drugs derived from the herbicide triazine is on the horizon and might provide some needed help. These drugs work differently than those currently available. Toltrazuril, one of the triazine derivatives, directly kills *S. neurona* in laboratory tests. Current therapy interferes with parasite multiplication, but relies on the horse's immune sytem to kill the parasite. Research in this area is in progress and should result in additional treatment choices in the near future.

Identification of the opossum as the definitive host has provided an unprecedented opportunity to study *S. neurona*. The infective form of the parasite (sporocyst) has been isolated from the opossum and used for direct study in the laboratory and in the field. The disease has been reproduced experimentally, which makes it possible to conduct controlled trials to evaluate the efficacy of potential vaccines and treatments. The door has been opened, and many investigators have entered the field of EPM research. Hopefully, this will help expedite development of effective methods of prevention and control of EPM.

SEARCHING FOR THE CAUSE

Rest assured, EPM has been with us for as long as opossums and horses have covered the same ground. However, few causes of equine neurologic disease were well differentiated prior to 1960. The terms "wobbler" and "spinal ataxia" (incoordination) were used as descriptive diagnoses that simply characterized the typical movement displayed by affected horses. In the early 1960s, two veterinary pathologists, Dr. John McGrath of the University of Pennsylvania and Dr. James Rooney of the University of Kentucky, independently described focal areas of hemorrhage in the central nervous system (CNS) of horses which had died due to neurologic disease. These areas had unique microscopic changes that distinguished them from CNS damage caused by other known equine neurologic diseases.

The initial EPM case in Kentucky was found in a Standardbred returning from tracks in the northeastern United States. Once the disease was recognized, it was found in many horses, including those which had not left Kentucky. Workers at the University of Kentucky reported 44 cases from late 1964-68. EPM initially was given descriptive names because protozoan parasites had not been observed in damaged areas of the CNS. It was first called "segmental myelitis" and later changed to "focal myelitis-encephalitis" to reflect focal or small scattered areas of damage in both the spinal cord (myelitis) and brain (encephalitis).

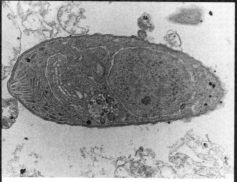

The *S. neurona* organism as seen under a transmission electron miograph.

Researchers speculated that the disease was caused by moldy feed. However, the microscopic damage was different from that found in moldy corn poisoning. Experiments conducted using various moldy feeds failed to reproduce EPM. The microscopic damage caused by EPM was similar to that caused by equine viral encephalomyelitis (Eastern, Western, and Venezuelan). However, consistent, recognizable differences were apparent. Interestingly, three different groups, led by Dr. John Cusick of the University of Illinois, Dr. J. P. Dubey of The Ohio State University, and Dr. Jill Beech of the University of Pennsylvania, independently reported the presence of protozoan parasites in characteristic areas of CNS damage in 1974.

Following some initial confusion regarding the identity of the parasite, it was shown that it was similar to, but definitely not, *Toxoplasma gondii*, a known pathogenic (harmful) protozoan of humans and many animals. Although the exact type of parasite was not known, Beech suggested that the drugs used to treat a similar protozoan affecting humans — toxoplasmosis — might be effective against the new EPM organism. Recognition of the parasite and the availability of treatment were the first major breakthroughs in EPM research since the disease had been described 12 years earlier.

In 1976, Dubey first suggested that the parasite was a

species of *Sarcocystis*. He conducted numerous experiments to identify the parasite and its life cycle. After moving to the U.S. Department of Agriculture's Agricultural Research Service, he and his co-workers, Dr. Stan Davis of the USDA-ARS and Dr. Dwight Bowman of Cornell University, cultured the parasite from an affected horse in 1990 and named it *S. neurona*. It had been 16 years since the last major breakthrough. Although this isolate soon died out, the experimental method had been established. A second isolate quickly was cultured from an equine spinal cord. This was followed by many isolations at the University of Kentucky and, subsequently, at the University of California at Davis.

During the late 1970s, Dr. Joe Mayhew and others at Cornell University carefully described many of the clinical aspects of the disease to help veterinarians differentiate EPM from other equine neurologic diseases. Unfortunately, no consistently reliable indicators of EPM could be found. During this period, Dr. Ron Fayer of the USDA-ARS and Dr. J. Carl Fox of Oklahoma State University each developed blood tests to detect antibodies to *Sarcocystis* in animals. Although quite different methods were used for each test, both immunoassays were based on *Sarcocystis* parasites isolated from cattle muscle. This meant that the tests were not specific for immunity to *S. neurona*.

That would not have been a problem if *S. neurona* had been the only *Sarcocystis* found in the horse. However, Dubey had estimated that 30% of horses in the United States also are infected with *Sarcocystis fayeri*, a relatively non-pathogenic parasite of the horse. Dubey discovered *S. fayeri* and named it in honor of Fayer, the first person to culture any *Sarcocystis*. This was a very significant event because it proved that *Sarcocystis* were protozoans, not fungi as previously believed.

DIAGNOSTIC TEST DEVELOPED

Cultured *S. neurona* merozoites were used to develop the parasite-specific EPM diagnostic test at the University of

Kentucky in 1991. The Western blot, or EPM test for blood or spinal fluid, was designed to differentiate exposure to *S. neurona* and *S. fayeri*. Initially, it was believed that the presence of *S. neurona*-specific antibodies in equine serum indicated that the horse had active EPM. This error was quickly recognized as exposure data were collected, showing that an average of 20% of normal horses on five farms tested positive. Although these data turned out to be well below those of larger surveys, they served to demonstrate that exposure to the parasite without clinical disease was common. Ultimately, cerebrospinal fluid (CSF) was found to provide valuable diagnostic information to differentiate exposure from active disease.

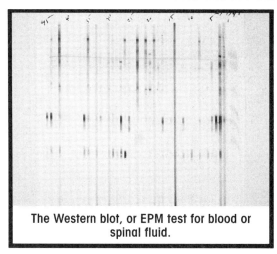
The Western blot, or EPM test for blood or spinal fluid.

Less than six months after the initial laboratory cultivation of *S. neurona*, the EPM test was fully operational, signaling the next major breakthrough. Both the initial culture and development of the EPM test were presented at a 1991 meeting of the American Association of Veterinary Parasitologists and the American Veterinary Medical Association. There, collaborations with Dr. Steve Reed of The Ohio State University and Dr. Alvin Gajadhar of Agriculture Canada were formed, which had a profound impact on EPM research at the University of Kentucky.

Reed and Lexington, Ky., veterinary internists Dr. Doug Byars and Dr. Bill Bernard contributed their time and case material to the project in which University of Kentucky pathologists also played an essential role. Soon, case material was arriving from many Central Kentucky veterinarians and eventually from throughout the Western hemisphere. Gajadhar of Agriculture Canada and University of Kentucky graduate students Dr. Clara Fenger and John Langemeier collaborated in the development of *S. neurona* DNA tests in 1994.

These results, in conjunction with field wildlife work done in collaboration with Dr. Judy Marteniuk and Dr. Jon Patterson of Michigan State University, resulted in identification of the opossum as the definitive host of *S. neurona* in early 1995. This work also led directly to the favorable comparison of *S. falcatula* from birds and *S. neurona* ribosomal genes by Dr. John Dame and Dr. Rob MacKay of the University of Florida in late 1995. Work at the University of Kentucky culminated in the most significant breakthrough to date — experimental reproduction of EPM in several horses in late 1995 and early 1996. This will permit direct study of host-parasite interaction critical for vaccine development and testing, as well as controlled studies to develop new treatments.

Although intense public pressure for answers has made progress seem slow, a series of research breakthroughs actually occurred in rapid succession. In fact, more has been learned about EPM in the last seven years than in the previous 30 years. Each discovery was essential for the next to occur. The field of EPM research is poised to explode. Strong public interest and general recognition of the scope of the problem have compelled granting agencies and corporate interests to fund more EPM research. Critical information and experimental material are readily available, making it possible for many investigators to enter this area of research. The next seven years hold great promise for understanding and ultimately overcoming EPM.

CHAPTER 1
What causes EPM?

EPM is caused by the parasite *Sarcocystis neurona*. All species of *Sarcocystis* are members of a vast group of single-celled animals known as protozoa. Most protozoans are microscopic, free-living organisms that do little harm. However, the genus *Sarcocystis* is made up of more than 100 individual species that are members of a large group (phylum) of parasitic protozoa known as apicomplexa. They depend on the cells of an animal host to survive and are unable to live indefinitely outside that host. Apicomplexans exist in many forms during the course of their reproductive cycle, but commonly exist in various merozoite stages — motile, banana-shaped bodies a few microns long (1 micron = 1/1,000,000 meters). The pointed end or apex of each merozoite is equipped with an elegantly formed system of fine tubules that allow it to penetrate host cell membranes. This is known as the apical complex and is the basis for membership in the phylum apicomplexa.

Sarcocystis have developed an incredibly ingenious scheme for survival. They have adapted to the predator-prey or scavenger-carrion relationships found among animals in nature. Individual *Sarcocystis* usually are very specific to single predator-prey or scavenger-carrion relationships and will not infect other hosts. By convention, parasitologists refer to the host that harbors sexually reproducing forms of a parasite as the definitive host of the parasite. Sexual reproduction occurs in cells lining the small intestine of the definitive host after the host has eaten infected prey or carrion. This form of reproduction is considered sexual because two gametes (similar to a sperm and an egg) produced from separate merozoites join to form a "fertilized egg" known as an oocyst. *Sarcocystis* oocysts are rounded microscopic bodies that consist of two oval sporocysts, each containing four banana-shaped sporozoites. Once fully formed, oocysts break free of intestinal lining cells and mix into the intestinal contents. *Sarcocystis* oocysts are unusually fragile and commonly rupture during the journey through the intestines. Individual sporocysts are found free in the feces of the definitive host. Sporocysts contaminate the environment and enter the food and water of the prey animal or intermediate host. They can survive for up to one year or more under temperate conditions and are resistant to common disinfectants such as chlorine bleach. Drying and prolonged freezing eventually kill them.

> **AT A GLANCE**
>
> - Equine protozoal myeloencephalitis (EPM) is caused by the parasite *Sarcocystis neurona*.
>
> - The opossum is the definitive host of *S. neurona*; horses become infected by ingesting water or food contaminated by opossum droppings.
>
> - The horse is a dead-end host for the parasite, meaning it cannot spread *S. neurona* to other horses or other animals.
>
> - The length of time between ingestion of the parasite and the onset of clinical signs can vary from less than 30 days to several years. Some horses can harbor the parasite without ever developing clinical signs.
>
> - The parasite can travel to any point in the central nervous system, including the brain and the spinal cord.

Once eaten by an appropriate intermediate host, sporocysts "hatch" or excyst in the small intestine. Motile sporozoites are released that quickly penetrate the intestine and enter specialized endothelial cells that line the interior surface of nearby blood vessels are released. Once inside the blood vessel wall, they begin rapid asexual division. More than 100 individual merozoites (tachyzoites) can bud from the nucleus of an original sporozoite to form a teaming mass of merozoites known as a meront (or schizont). The endothelial cell eventually bursts, showering the bloodstream with new merozoites. Each merozoite is carried to another endothelial cell and the process is repeated at least once more. Thus the parasite has managed to amplify dramatically the initial infection and enhance its chances for survival. However, some infections can become rapidly fatal if a large dose of sporocysts has been ingested by the intermediate host.

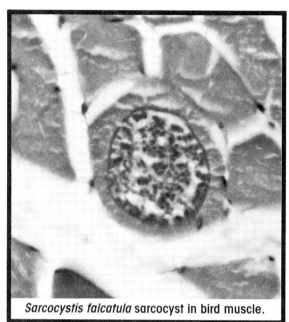

Sarcocystis falcatula sarcocyst in bird muscle.

After the last round of rapid asexual division, merozoites typically enter individual muscle cells and begin to divide very slowly. A cyst wall forms around them to create a sarcocyst in the muscle of the intermediate host. Mature or infective sarcocysts generally are present in the muscle two months following sporocyst ingestion. Sarcocysts grow slowly and can remain in the muscle of the intermediate host for extended periods, up to several years, without causing any disturbance. Sarcocysts of some species grow so large that they become visible to the naked eye. Perhaps, you have seen *S. rileyi* in ducks or geese. They look like grains of rice embedded in the muscle fibers. Although rare, mild to severe myositis (muscle inflammation) can develop early in the course of heavy infections with various species.

Sarcocysts of individual *Sarcocystis* are infective for a

narrow range of definitive hosts. The relationship is somewhat less restrictive than the sporocyst-intermediate host interaction, but it still is quite limited. For example, *S. cruzi* sporocysts infect cattle but not other ruminants (sheep, deer, elk), while *S. cruzi* sarcocysts infect all canids (dog, wolf, coyote, fox), as well as the racoon. *Sarcocystis muris* sporocysts infect mice, but not other rodents, while *S. muris* sarcocysts infect all felids. *Sarcocystis falcatula* sporocysts are quite unusual because they infect a wide variety of birds.

Once infected muscle has been eaten and digested, individual merozoites (bradyzoites) are released into the small intestine of the definitive host. They quickly enter intestinal lining cells and form "male" and "female" gametes as the process of sexual reproduction begins once again. Sporocysts can appear in the feces of the definitive host a little more than a week following the ingestion of infected meat.

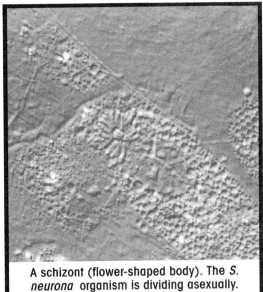

A schizont (flower-shaped body). The *S. neurona* organism is dividing asexually.

Sarcocystis fayeri and two other *Sarcocystis* use this life cycle to alternate between horses and canids. Infection rarely results in clinical signs, but a few cases of severe myositis have been reported in the veterinary literature. Unlike *S. fayeri*, merozoites of *S. neurona* enter the central nervous system (CNS), not muscle. The mode of entry into the CNS is not known. It is assumed that they directly penetrate the blood-brain barrier, a layer of tightly joined endothelial cells lining CNS blood vessels. It also is possible that merozoites enter the

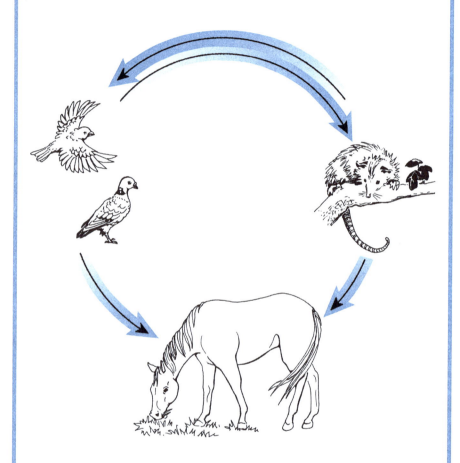

The life cycle of the EPM parasite

Birds carry the parasite in their muscles; opossums eat dead birds and pass the parasite in their feces, where it is picked up when horses eat or drink. It is also thought that birds can contaminate the environment.

CNS hidden within white blood cells that routinely pass through the blood-brain barrier. Some have suggested that merozoites leave blood vessels in other parts of the body, enter adjacent peripheral nerves, and migrate up the nerves to reach the CNS. This seems highly unlikely. Intracellular merozoites of this stage divide rapidly; meronts developing at distant sites should produce local inflammation in peripheral nerves. The pain associated with the inflammation could be blocked with local anesthetic. Certainly, horses often have multiple problems, but one of the hallmarks of EPM diagnosis is apparent lameness that cannot be blocked locally.

Once inside the CNS, sarcocysts fail to form and merozoites continue rapidly dividing into large meronts inside nerve cells and other cell types in the horse's brain and spinal cord. Merozoites are not infective for definitive hosts, so the infection does not spread if the horse dies and is eaten. Horses are accidental or aberrant, dead-end hosts of *S. neurona*. Once sporocysts have excysted in the horse's small intestine, the parasite cannot be passed to another host.

There has been some speculation that pregnant mares might pass *S. neurona* to their unborn foals, but that has never been confirmed. It is worth considering because prenatal transmission of *Sarcocystis* is known to occur in many appropriate intermediate hosts. For example, *S. cruzi* has caused a number of abortion "storms" in cattle. *Neospora caninum*, another apicomplexan protozoa, is a major cause of abortion in dairy cattle in California. It recently was cultured from a horse in California with protozoal encephalitis. Equine neosporosis apparently plays an insignificant role in EPM, but a few general infections have been reported, including an aborted equine fetus.

We now know that the opossum is the definitive host of *S. neurona* and that horses become infected by ingesting food or water contaminated by infected opossum droppings. Sporocysts can be disseminated further in a variety of ways.

Birds attracted to seeds or bugs feeding on opossum feces have been shown to pass sporocysts in their feces. An unexplored method of dissemination involves a type of grain or harvest mite. These microsopic insects feed on a wide variety of organic matter in soil and are an essential part of the life cycle of equine tapeworms. They ingest tapeworm eggs from horse feces that subsequently hatch and develop into an infective intermediate stage called a cysticercoid.

Horses become infected as they graze on pasture or eat mites with hay. Mites feed in the top layer of soil, but migrate up blades of grass during the day. Tapeworms mostly are viewed as nuisance parasites, and their control in equine deworming programs often is overlooked. Consequently, a high percentage of horses are infected. Perhaps a similar scenario partially is responsible for the high exposure rate of *S. neurona* among horses.

The length of time between sporocyst ingestion and the onset of clinical signs, called the incubation period, is highly variable. Recent experimental studies at the University of Kentucky demonstrated that clinical signs of EPM can develop less than 30 days after sporocyst ingestion. It also is known that horses shipped to countries without EPM can harbor *S. neurona* for months or even years prior to the onset of clinical signs. The parasite's location during this period is not known, but it seems likely that it persists in low numbers in the CNS. Infection has not been found anywhere else in the horse's body.

The other half of the *S. neurona* life cycle is less certain. Initial molecular and immunologic comparisons suggested that *S. neurona* was actually *S. falcatula*. It has been known since 1978 that *S. falcatula* cycles between opossums and various birds. The parasite originally was named when small, but visible, sarcocysts were observed in the muscles of a rose-breasted grosbeak more than 100 years ago. Additional molecular evidence and transmission studies in birds suggest that *S.*

falcatula might contain a number of subspecies or strains. If pathogenic and non-pathogenic strains prove to be sufficiently different, it is possible that the name *S. neurona* will be retained to recognize this group as a unique species.

Birds become infected with *S. falcatula* by ingesting sporocysts from opossum feces. A recent survey of opposums in Central Kentucky found sporocysts in more than one-third of the animals examined. A study done in Maryland in the early 1970s found that more than 90% of adult grackles were infected with *S. falcatula* sarcocysts. Common song and pest birds are somewhat resistant to clinical infection. However, many exotic birds are highly susceptible to overwhelming pulmonary infection and might die before sarcocysts have formed in their muscles. Chickens, turkeys, ducks, and geese are completely resistant to *S. falcatula* infection. Sporocysts can be transported to birds (and horses) in or on various bugs and insects attracted to opossum feces. Interestingly, a fatal *S. falcatula* epidemic among parakeets in a Florida aviary was stopped by introducing flightless chickens to control a rampant roach population. Another study demonstrated that sporocysts stick to the feet and legs of flies after landing on the feces of an infected definitive host.

EPIDEMIOLOGY AND RISK FACTORS

Epidemiology refers to the study of the health and disease of a population rather than an individual. Epidemiologic studies gather information about a population to discover factors that increase the risk of spreading and maintaining a particular disease among the individuals of the population. Ultimately, understanding the risk factors for the population directly benefits the individual as well.

Several epidemiologic studies have been done to evaluate EPM over the years. A major limiting factor associated with earlier studies was the reliance on postmortem examination to confirm the diagnosis of EPM. The only horses evaluated were those so severely affected that they failed to survive. Therefore, only a small proportion of the horses with EPM were included in the studies. In addition, regional bias was introduced due to the variable cost of postmortem examination and the extent of the CNS evaluation performed at each facility. Some state diagnostic laboratories provide free services, while others charge hundreds of dollars for an examination that includes the entire CNS. Removal of the brain and spinal cord of an adult horse is very labor-intensive. Partial removal is much easier to perform, but several feet of valuable tissue are lost. It also is very difficult for veterinarians in the field to submit more than the brain and the first few inches of spinal cord for examination. Despite these shortcomings, retrospective studies of postmortem data have provided a great deal of useful information.

The type of information usually gathered includes age, breed, and sex of horse; location; number of horses affected; number dead; and a brief clinical history. Clinical histories include duration of illness, clinical signs, treatment, and response to treatment.

EPM CAN STRIKE ALMOST ANY HORSE

The American College of Veterinary Internal Medicine sponsored an EPM workshop at its 1988 annual meeting. Veterinary pathologists, parasitologists, and clinicians gathered from across North America. The workshop was based on 364 postmortem confirmed cases of EPM from veterinary diagnostic laboratories in California, Florida, Illinois, Kentucky, New York, Ohio, Oklahoma, Pennsylvania, Texas, and Ontario, Canada. Representatives from each institution presented a review of cases accumulated over an average of six years (range of four to 12 years). Affected horses ranged in age from two months to 19 years. The majority of the affected horses were young; more than 60% were four years old or less.

The most commonly affected breeds in rank

order were Thoroughbreds, Standardbreds, and Quarter Horses, but most other breeds and ponies were affected. No preference was found based on sex, geographic location, or time of year. The percent of all neurologic disease diagnosed at each facility due to EPM was not reported. However, postmortem studies at Cornell University and the University of Kentucky have reported rates of 25% and 9%, respectively. A recent clinical retrospective (with or without postmortem) done at The Ohio State University from 1991-94 found that 25% of all spinal ataxia was due to EPM. Although many other neurologic diseases are present, EPM is without doubt the most common neurologic disease among horses in North America today.

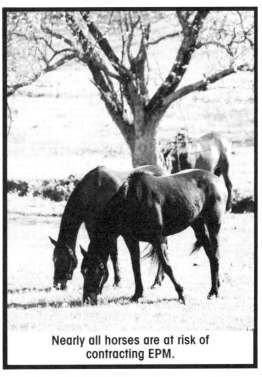

Nearly all horses are at risk of contracting EPM.

Results from the 1988 workshop generally agreed with those of a four-year retrospective study done at the University of Kentucky's Livestock Disease Diagnostic Center from 1988-91. At Kentucky, 60% of affected horses were three years old or less. In addition, a seasonal trend was noted as more cases were diagnosed in the spring and summer. Other regional studies done at Cornell University and the University of Pennsylvania found that Standardbreds were more frequently affected than Thoroughbreds even though fewer Standardbreds were received for examination. The

Pennsylvania study also found that young male horses were most often affected, but this was attributed to the over-representation of this group among the racehorse population that dominated its clinical practice. One final difference from the ACVIM study should be noted.

While that study was national in scope, a number of arid western states were not in attendance. That was because very little EPM occurs in these states. Therefore, the fact that no geographic predilection was found is not too surprising.

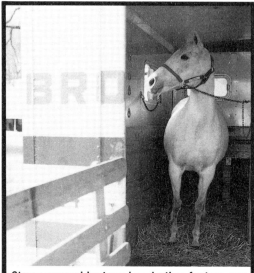
Stress caused by travel and other factors can make the immune system vulnerable.

Although age and breed certainly seem to be factors, all horses are susceptible to *S. neurona*. Management factors associated with racing must be considered. Young horses are placed into rigorous training and competition schedules which often require thousands of miles of travel during the season. Although racehorses generally receive excellent care, physical and environmental stresses are known to affect the immune system negatively. EPM frequently has been associated with known causes of stress such as shipping and pregnancy. Initial disease and clinical relapse also have been associated with heavy work and steroid administration. Steroids are excellent anti-inflammatory drugs that also result in some suppression of the immune response. Low levels are produced naturally in the body and are essential for life. Increased release of steroids during periods of physical or environmental stress is partly to blame for immune suppression. Many veterinary clinicians and researchers believe that stress is a major risk factor for the development of clinical signs of EPM.

An issue related to immune status is genetic predisposition to susceptibility. This topic has received only anecdotal consideration at best. Certainly, some individuals in any population will be more susceptible to a particular infectious agent than others. Internal factors that control the immune response are passed genetically from parents to their offspring. However, there is no hard evidence to suggest that affected stallions or mares pass any increased susceptibility to EPM to their foals. While this may occur, the lack of obvious evidence suggests that other risk factors are much more important.

DEVELOPING EPM REQUIRES EXPOSURE FIRST

Before stress can influence the clinical onset of EPM, horses must first be exposed to *S. neurona*. The number of parasites ingested is a known risk factor for the development of clinical sarcocystosis in many intermediate hosts. *Sarcocystis cruzi* in cattle provide an excellent example. It has been demonstrated experimentally that small numbers of sporocysts produce no obvious signs of infection in cattle. In fact, it has been estimated that all cattle in the United States eventually become exposed to *Sarcocystis*. Like EPM, relatively few exposures result in clinical disease. Larger numbers of *S. cruzi* sporocysts produce myositis, chronic wasting, and abortion, while even larger doses result in widespread areas of inflammation, anemia, and death. By comparison, extremely large numbers of sporocysts were required to produce EPM experimentally in horses. Although none of the horses were severely affected, low doses were not effective.

The EPM blood test has been used to estimate the prevalence of *S. neurona* antibodies in serum (seroprevalence) among horses in several states. The first large study included 40 randomly selected farms from the "Bluegrass" region of Central Kentucky. Blood samples from more than 500 horses were tested, which resulted in an exposure rate above 45%. A similar exposure rate was found in a study of 117 horses randomly selected from all Thoroughbred farms in Chester County, Pennsylvania.

A somewhat different experimental approach was used to estimate seroprevalence in Oregon. Twenty-one veterinarians, distributed evenly across the state, randomly collected 334 blood samples from client horses. An average exposure rate of 45% was found. However, when sample results were evaluated based on geographic location, a fascinating discovery was made. Four regions were created by dividing the state longitudinally into four equal sections from east to west. Seroprevalence dramatically increased from a low of 22% in the arid eastern region to a high of 65% in the humid west. Interestingly, these results mirror the location of the opossum population in Oregon. Another study of 300 horses was done using blood samples from wild horses caught in Utah. Seroprevalence was less than 1%. Apparently, opossums and sporocysts both do poorly in hot, dry climates.

> **AT A GLANCE**
>
> - EPM can affect any breed, but one major study found that the most commonly affected breeds were Thoroughbreds, Standardbreds, and Quarter Horses in that order.
>
> - Young horses are affected more often than older horses, but older horses are exposed more frequently.
>
> - Stress is thought to trigger clinical onset in some horses.
>
> - Horses must be exposed to the parasite before they can develop EPM.
>
> - Blood tests can confirm exposure to EPM, but a positive blood test does not mean that a horse has the disease.

Two seroprevalence studies have been done using blood samples randomly selected from blood samples submitted for Coggins testing. A current Coggins test is required for most equine events and interstate travel. Some argue that this mobility introduces too much error for accurate analysis of exposure rate based on Coggins samples. Undoubtedly, travel does affect the results. However, samples submitted for Coggins testing provide a readily available resource that is very well defined. Totally random sampling of all horses in a large area is labor intensive and cost prohibitive.

The largest EPM study using Coggins blood samples was

done in Ohio, where more than 1,000 samples were selected. The excellent information included with the samples revealed that submissions were present from 81 of 88 Ohio counties and virtually all breeds found in the state. The average exposure rate was almost 54%. However, a significant difference in exposure rate was found between the northeast (45%) and the southwest regions (62%) of the state. This was found to be associated with the number of days below freezing in each region. As the number of days below freezing increased, the seroprevalence decreased. Just as the Oregon study confirmed the effect of arid conditions on sporocyst survival, the Ohio study provided practical confirmation that sporocysts are susceptible to prolonged freezing. This result also helps validate the use of Coggins blood samples for seroprevalence studies.

A similar study was done at Colorado State University using more than 600 Coggins samples. Although the results have not been fully analyzed, the seroprevalence was under 35%. This result coincides with the lower exposure rate found in the arid regions of eastern Oregon.

OLDER HORSES EXPOSED MORE OFTEN

A direct correlation between age and seroprevalence was a recurrent theme among the seroprevalence studies that were fully analyzed. The exposure rate consistently increased with age. This is not too surprising, given that older horses have had more time to become exposed. However, the degree of increase is both startling and informative. In Pennsylvania (state average 45%), horses less than one year old had an exposure rate of 15% and horses older than 14 were exposed 61% of the time. Similarly, in Oregon (state average 45%), horses less than one year old had an exposure rate of 15%, while horses older than 15 were positive 64% of the time. Aged horses in the Ohio study (state average 54%) reached the highest exposure rate. Horses less than six years old had an exposure rate of 46%, while 82% of horses older than 16 tested positive. Undoubtedly, horses are exposed to *S. neurona* repeatedly. If the interval between significant exposures is not prolonged, antibody production is boosted and the horse could remain positive for an indefinite period.

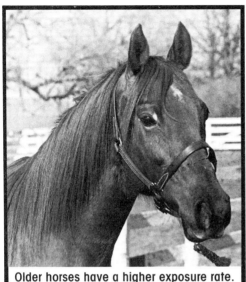

Older horses have a higher exposure rate.

We already know that horses can remain seropositive for years without developing clinical signs. It is also readily apparent that the parasite can be harbored in the horse for months, or even years before causing clinical disease. This has been demonstrated by the two-year delay in development of clinical disease in horses shipped to countries where EPM is not known to occur. Unfortunately, these cases were reported before the advent of the EPM test, so information regarding the presence of antibody in serum or spinal fluid is not available.

RESEARCH IN PROGRESS

Researchers at several institutions are continuing various molecular, immunologic, and transmission studies to resolve the issues surrounding the relationship between *S. neurona* and *S. falcatula*. Molecular comparisons have moved to the sequence analysis of multiple genes and the incorporation of alternative techniques for comparison of DNA. A major drawback has been the availability of pure material to study. Parasites cultured from individual horses have been considered a single strain of *S. neurona*. However, sporocysts harvested from laboratory-raised opossums were derived after the opossums had eaten birds infected with mixed populations of sarcocysts. Researchers must produce a number of clonal populations of *S. falcatula* derived from single sporocysts or sarcocysts to determine if opossums and birds share the same parasite or several very similar ones.

Ultimately, parasite populations derived from single merozoites, sporocysts, or sarcocysts also will be necessary to make accurate immunologic comparisons and to conduct meaningful transmission studies. At the University of Kentucky, three opossum sporocyst isolates were excysted, cultured, and compared by immunoblot analysis using serum and spinal fluid from horses with EPM. The results of these studies demonstrated that the opossum sporozoites were virtually identical to merozoites cultured from horses. Other investigators also are attempting immunologic comparison of cultured sporozoites.

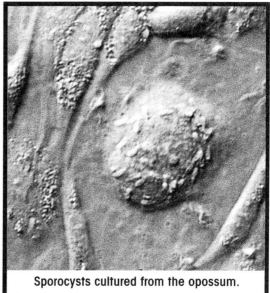

Sporocysts cultured from the opossum.

Interestingly, only two of the three sporozoite cultures tested positive using an *S. neurona*-specific polymerase chain reaction (PCR) DNA test. This suggests a difference in the DNA sequence of the small ribosomal subunit gene used to develop the PCR test. However, the mixed nature of the sporocyst population cultured for these studies precludes definite conclusions. Other researchers have also reported sequence variation in this gene and related ones.

EPM was reproduced experimentally using sporocysts from feral opossums. This proved that the opossum is the definitive host of *S. neurona*, but said little about the identity of the intermediate host. Sporocysts from the same stock given to horses also were given to uninfected sparrows. All of the birds developed sarcocystosis and were fed to laboratory-raised opossums. The opossums produced sporocysts, proving that *S. falcatula* was present in the inoculum given to the horses.

However, another *Sarcocystis* could have been present as well. These sporocysts then were used in an experiment designed to determine if *S. neurona* and at least some isolates of *S. falcatula* were identical. EPM was not reproduced. This could mean that the sporocysts responsible for producing EPM do not cycle through sparrows. They could cycle through other birds and still be considered *S. falcatula,* or they might use an entirely different intermediate host. Unfortunately, the sporocysts used in this study were six to eight months old when the experimental infections were attempted. Although the sporocysts appeared normal, it is possible that the effective or viable doses were well below the actual numbers of sporocysts given. This study will be repeated, preferably using clonally derived sporocysts.

Transmission studies being done at other institutions (University of Florida, University of California) include administration of opossum sporocysts to horses and cultured *S. neurona* and *S. falcatula* merozoites to birds. Researchers hope to use these methodologies to identify the relationship between the parasites.

A large multicenter prospective study has been proposed by The Ohio State University. If funded, researchers there will coordinate the collection of detailed information from 800 EPM cases at eight centers across the United States. This project would provide invaluable insight into the major risk factors for EPM. It should also identify an optimal treatment regimen. Ohio State also is working on a comprehensive retrospective study of more than 400 neurologic cases that will provide additional analysis of risk factors, diagnostic testing, and treatment effectiveness.

Michigan State University is conducting a regional prospective study to identify risk factors of EPM. Additional seroprevalence studies also are in progress in several states.

CHAPTER 2
What Are the Clinical Signs of EPM?

A brief review of the horse's nervous system will help provide a more complete understanding of the clinical signs of EPM. The basic subunit of the nervous system is the nerve cell or neuron. Neurons conduct nerve impulses, which form the communication network for the entire body. Neurons are "terminally differentiated" cells. In other words, they are so advanced that they can no longer divide. Once damaged beyond repair, individual neurons are lost forever. However, there are more than enough neurons built into the nervous system. They operate in interconnected groups, so that if one neuron dies, the function it performed is not necessarily lost. Neurons extend a few short processes and one long process called an axon, or nerve fiber, to communicate. Information is transmitted to and from the central nervous system through a continuous succession of neurons and axons, which form nerves.

There are three types of neurons: sensory, interneuron, and motor. Sensory neurons are located outside the CNS and gather information about the body and environment. The CNS is bombarded constantly by incoming signals from the axons of sensory nerves. Some neurons actually provide inhibitory input. Without these inhibitory signals for down regulation, the brain would be unable to function. Strychnine poisoning depresses inhibitory neurons and results in widespread muscular contraction due to the loss of down regulation.

Interneurons are located within the CNS. Their function is to relay information from the sensory neurons and other interneurons back to motor neurons. Motor neurons are located in the CNS and send signals via axons to all the muscles and glands throughout the body.

Motor nerve signals initiate action in muscles and glands and provide constant low-level stimulation, which maintains muscle tone.

The brain processes the sensory information received from the rest of the body and transmits signals which reflect deci-

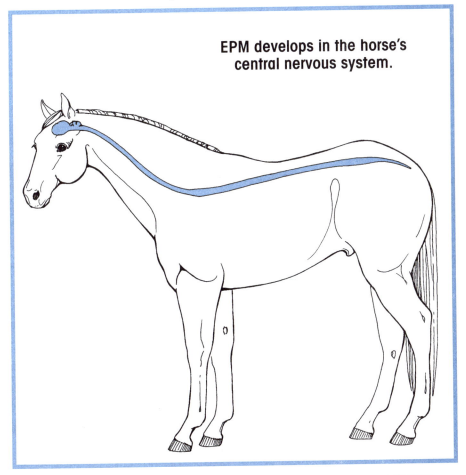

EPM develops in the horse's central nervous system.

sions to initiate action. The brain, essentially a large mass of interconnected neurons and axons, must respond properly to all stimuli for the body to function normally. Specific groups of neurons in well-defined areas of the brain cooperate to perform the specific functions necessary for life. Twelve cranial nerves originate from discrete neuron groupings or nuclei in the brainstem, which control most functions of the head and neck. Every body function is controlled by the CNS: heartbeat, temperature regulation, intestinal motility, breathing, body movement, emotion, etc. Damage to specific areas results in very predictable clinical signs.

The horse's spinal cord is a soft, white, cylindrical structure that runs from the base of the skull to the small of the back. Its diameter varies from one-half inch to more than an inch as it travels inside the vertebral column toward the tail. Location along the vertebral column is designated by region: cervical (neck), thoracic (chest), lumbar (mid-back), sacral (lower back), coccygeal (tail), and vertebral number within the region (C1-7, T1-18, L1-6, S1-5, Cy1-21). When cut in cross-section, the spinal cord is oval and reveals a butterfly-shaped gray area (gray matter) surrounded by white matter. Gray matter is made up of neurons (interneurons and motor neurons), while white matter consists of axons from sensory (asending) and motor (desending) neurons.

CRANIAL NERVES AND FUNCTIONS

No.	Name	Function
I.	Olfactory	Sense of smell
II.	Optic	Sight
III.	Occulomotor	Iris (pupil constriction), eye muscles, upper eyelid
IV.	Trochlear	Eye muscles
V.	Trigeminal	Jaw muscles; Sensory to face, mouth, and teeth
VI.	Abducens	Eye muscles
VII.	Facial	Facial muscles; Sensory to first 2/3 of tongue
VIII.	Vestibulocochlear	Hearing and equilibrium
IX.	Glossopharyngeal	Tongue, throat, and palate muscles; Sensory to throat and last 1/3 of tongue
X.	Vagus	Organ muscles (lungs, heart, intestines), palate muscle; Sensory to throat and lungs
XI.	Spinal Accessory	Throat and shoulder muscles
XII.	Hypoglossal	Tongue

Spinal nerves exit the spinal cord at each vertebral joint. Spinal nerves are formed by thousands of sensory and motor axons. Except for the cranial nerves, all the nerves supplying the periphery (rest of the body) ultimately branch from spinal nerves. Damage to the root or starting point of a particular spinal nerve within the spinal cord results in very specific loss of function(s) controlled by that nerve and its branches. This often includes the loss or enhancement of specific reflexes, which can be useful for diagnosis.

INFECTION, INFLAMMATION, AND CLINICAL DISEASE

Sarcocystis neurona can strike the CNS anywhere along the brain or spinal cord. It attacks gray and white matter with similar frequency. It most often infects several specific areas at once (multifocal) and rarely produces diffuse or widespread damage. EPM is a highly variable clinical disease. Depending on the location and number of parasites present, individual infections might manifest insidiously, producing very subtle signs, or might strike with incredible speed, resulting in very dramatic loss of function.

Although it is unusual, the inflammation and swelling caused by *S. neurona* infection can become rapidly life-threatening. Since the CNS is encased in bone, there is very little room to accommodate swelling. The resultant pressure compromises the blood supply to the CNS, which is critical for the survival of nervous tissue. Neurons are so specialized that they have very little energy reserve. Consequently, they have a very high oxygen requirement and die within sec-

> **AT A GLANCE**
>
> - Inflammation of the central nervous system results when the horse's immune system fights the invading parasites.
>
> - Inflammation and swelling caused by *S. neurona* infection sometimes can lead to a life-threatening situation.
>
> - Clinical signs of EPM are directly related to the site of specific lesions in the brain or spinal cord.
>
> - Clinical signs can range from seizures and depression to loss of sight, hearing, taste, touch, and coordination.

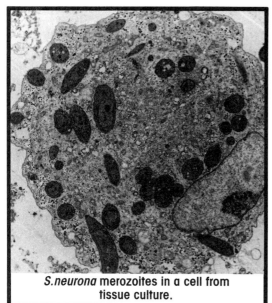

S. *neurona* merozoites in a cell from tissue culture.

onds if this demand is not met. This is how a horse can appear normal loading onto a trailer in the morning and be unable to walk off that afternoon.

When the merozoites of the parasite enter the nervous system of the horse, a battle ensues. The horse's immune system is battling the parasite, resulting in inflammation and other responses. It is ironic that while the body is fighting off an invader, the battle itself can become life-threatening to the horse.

One aspect of this battle is a dramatic increase in the porosity of the horse's blood-brain barrier. A rapid influx of fluid, serum components, and white blood cells occurs, which is required to win the battle against the invaders. However, there is not a corresponding increase in outflow. The resultant disruption of normal CNS architecture and increased pressure restrict normal blood flow to the immediate area. Interference with oxygen availability results in rapid neuronal death. In addition, toxic products released to kill parasites and substances inadvertently released from dead and dying cells further contribute to the damage. At postmortem, the damaged areas, called lesions, typically appear as focal areas of hemorrhage and swelling on the cut surface of the spinal cord.

Elimination of parasites removes the stimulus for these events and damaged areas eventually are cleaned up by specialized cells, which multiply for this purpose. Lost neurons cannot be replaced, but gradually damaged areas will heal, leaving characteristic scars. Clinical signs caused by pressure, without widespread neuronal death, should subside. Neurologic deficits due to the death of neurons or axons can return only if a sufficient number of appropriate neurons remain to compensate for their loss. The repair and recovery process can take months, particularly when some parasites persist. At present, we do not know if this battle in the CNS is waged routinely following ingestion of sporocysts, or if merozoites are eliminated before they cross the blood-brain barrier. It seems likely that both scenarios occur on a fairly routine basis. The emergence of clinical signs on any given day would simply depend on which direction the dynamic balance between the parasite burden and host response is tipped.

SIGNS OF EPM CAN VARY WIDELY

It now should be evident that the clinical signs of EPM are directly related to the location of specific lesions in the brain or

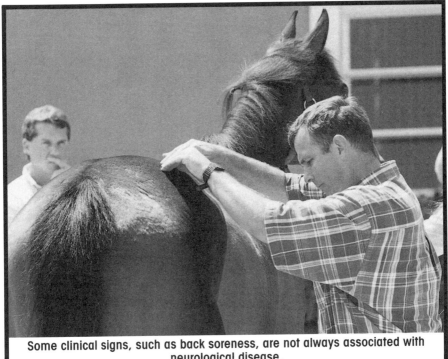

Some clinical signs, such as back soreness, are not always associated with neurological disease.

spinal cord. Because the disease is multifocal, or can affect more than one area at the same time, a wide range of neurologic deficits can occur in various combinations within any individual. Damage to the brain might result in behavioral or cognitive deficits unique to the cerebral cortex (seizures, depression, memory loss) or might produce signs attributable to brainstem damage (loss of sight, hearing, balance, smell, taste, touch, coordination; difficulty eating; personality change). Due to the integration or processing of all information in the brain, brain damage might mimic direct sensory (coordination) and/or motor (muscle wasting, weakness, paralysis) pathway damage to the spinal cord or peripheral nerves.

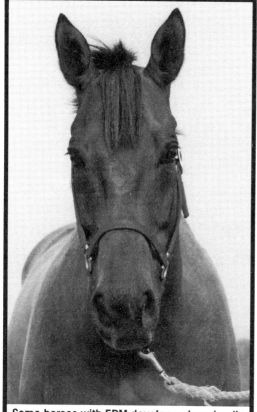

Some horses with EPM develop a drooping lip or other signs of facial paralysis.

Many authors have commented in the veterinary and lay literature about the vast array of common to bizarre clincal signs associated with EPM. I think most would agree that ataxia (incoordination) of one or both rear limbs is recognized more frequently than any other clinical sign of EPM. If both back legs are affected, one is usually more severely affected than the other because separate areas of infection are responsible for impairing the function of each limb. Clinicians often refer to this as "asymmetric posterior ataxia," with it being more severe or lateralizing to the left or right side of the horse depending on which is more severely affected. Typically, the underlying cause of this problem is a discrete lesion(s) involving sensory axons in the spinal cord past the second thoracic vertebra (T2). However, lesions of the brain, brain stem, or inner ear also might cause ataxia. Sensory pathway damage to the spinal cord up to and including T2 involves the front legs, but often includes one or both back legs due to lesions affecting sensory axons supplying the rear limbs. Nerves serving the front limbs branch from the spinal cord before T2, and those serving the rear limbs branch after T2.

Damage to the motor pathways of the spinal cord might result in weakness (truncal sway, toe dragging), paralysis, and atrophy (wasting) of the muscle(s) served by the affected nerves. Muscle atrophy most commonly occurs over the hips or shoulders, but rarely does it become widespread. Many of these clinical signs often accompany ataxia. It becomes easy to appreciate why a horse with multiple lesions in gray and white matter of the spinal cord becomes ataxic. Loss of sensory and motor nerve input diminishes proprioception (sense of limb position) and the horse's ability to initiate movement.

Lesions occurring at the sacral end of the spinal cord (L6-S2) frequently result in the loss of muscle tone in the anus and tail, as well as loss of skin sensation in the area. Affected horses might dribble urine due to partial or complete bladder paralysis. Rectal paralysis also occurs, which can lead to colic due to impaction.

> **AT A GLANCE**
>
> - Ataxia, or incoordination of one or both rear limbs, is recognized more frequently than any other clinical sign of EPM.
>
> - Horses with EPM sometimes have a proprioceptive deficit, meaning their awareness of limb placement is compromised.
>
> - Muscle atrophy sometimes accompanies ataxia and commonly occurs over the hips or shoulders.
>
> - When EPM strikes the brain, infection can lead to behavioral changes.
>
> - Subtle neurological signs can signal EPM. They might include bucking, high head carriage, back soreness, inappropriate lead changes, and unequal stride length.
>
> - Each case of EPM is different and unpredictable, adding to the confusion and debate over the disease.

Subtle signs associated with mild CNS lesions apparently are more common than generally appreciated (or accepted). It seems reasonable to assume that a gradual (or occasionally rapid) progression of clinical signs results as lesions become worse and infection spreads. At some point, the effects of infection become recognizable. Part of the controversy surrounding EPM is due to the difficulty in detecting subtle signs, then attributing them to EPM. For example, many diseases result in training problems and/or poor athletic performance. While it is clear that EPM is certainly one of these, the real question becomes "how often?" It is not always readily apparent that some clinical signs are associated with neurologic disease at all. Many are more often associated with various causes of lameness, muscle soreness, and behavioral problems. Those described include frequent bucking, head tossing, high head carriage, back soreness, inappropriate lead changes, unequal stride length, and other subtle gait abnormalities.

The most compelling reason to consider EPM when these clinical signs are observed is the growing body of evidence provided by horses which have progressed to obvious neurologic disease that either responded to treatment or were confirmed by postmortem examination.

At the same time, many horses exhibit these signs and do not appear to progress. Did they have EPM and fight it off without treatment? Did they ever have EPM at all? It is very difficult to determine. In addition, it is important to realize that neurologic disease can result in musculoskeletal injuries and true lameness. All of these factors add to the confusion and debate over EPM and create quite a dilemma for veterinary practitioners. It becomes that much more difficult to decide when to place EPM on the list of possible causes of various clinical problems.

One of the most important points to remember is that EPM produces highly variable clinical disease. Each individual case is unique and unpredictable. Many of the questions regarding the how, when, why, and where of EPM do not have good answers. It is unrealistic to expect the attending veterinarian to provide definitive answers. Ultimately, the knowledge and experience of the attending veterinarian provide the best hope for a rapid, accurate diagnosis. The use of various diagnostic aids often is helpful and will be discussed in subsequent chapters.

CHAPTER 3
How is EPM Diagnosed?

A veterinarian's ability to make the correct diagnosis is always enhanced by a thorough, accurate clinical history of the affected horse and others at the same location. Important clues about the cause of the disorder might be revealed. In addition to age, breed, and sex, the veterinarian will need to know the vaccination and de-worming schedule, feeding history, changes in appetite, any behavioral changes, the rate of onset and duration of any clinical signs, and all recent changes in the horse's environment or management.

A thorough neurologic examination is the single most important part of an effective diagnostic plan for EPM. Musculoskeletal injuries (muscle, tendon, ligament, or bone) occur much more commonly than EPM. Therefore, the importance of differentiating lameness from neurologic deficits is critical. Musculoskeletal injuries might result from underlying neurologic disorders, making the recognition of concurrent neurologic deficits more difficult. In many cases, this differentiation can be made easily, but unusual or mildly affected horses can be very difficult to assess.

The use of local anesthetics to perform nerve blocks is

UNDERSTANDING EPM

often helpful. Horses return to normal following a nerve block only when the problem is local. Clinical signs due to central nervous system involvement are unaffected by local or regional nerve blocks. The horse will continue to appear "lame." The multifocal nature of CNS damage due to EPM is often useful for differentiation from lameness, as well as other neurologic disorders. Clinical evidence of neurologic damage at multiple sites within the CNS is highly suggestive of EPM. This is especially helpful when improvement or complete function has returned to an individual limb following a nerve block, but other limbs fail to respond.

> **AT A GLANCE**
>
> - A thorough neurological exam is crucial in effectively diagnosing EPM.
> - All other disorders should be ruled out first.
> - Other equine diseases can affect the horse's neurological system.
> - Laboratory tests can help differentiate EPM from other diseases.
> - Development of accurate diagnostic tests for EPM is continuing.

After recognizing that a neurologic disease is at work, the veterinarian must differentiate the particular disorder(s) responsible. Again, a thorough neurologic exam is of the utmost importance. Careful consideration of exam results and history should suggest a short list of differential diagnoses that might require additional diagnostic testing. The chart that appears at the end of this chapter is an example of an excellent neurologic examination form developed at The Ohio State University. Hopefully, a thorough discussion of this form and the underlying reasons for its configuration will help illustrate the complexity of neurologic diseases in general and provide a greater understanding of EPM.

The basis of the neurologic exam form can be found in the neuroanatomical discussion in the previous chapter. A methodical, systematic analysis of neural pathways, starting with the head and ending at the tail, has been outlined. Behavioral abnormalities (depression, belligerence, loss of appetite), seizures, or blindness might indicate brain lesions. Reflexes involving the cranial and other peripheral nerves are evaluated on both sides of the body. Loss of skin sensation is evaluated and mapped if present. Differentiation between the loss of skin sensation and the ability to feel pain is useful to help determine the extent of damage. Many muscles and muscle groups are assessed for tone and strength and compared from side to side. Movement is evaluated in all directions and under different circumstances to evaluate sensory and motor innervation. Standing limb position or placement is tested to further assess proprioception and to help localize CNS damage.

DIFFERENTIAL DIAGNOSIS

Although EPM is the most commonly diagnosed equine neurologic disease in the Western Hemisphere, many other neurologic disorders affect horses as well. Accurate interpretation of neurologic exam findings and clinical history requires a thorough understanding of these disorders. A discussion of the most common of these follows in approximate order of occurrence in North America. Regional differences in frequency are common. Consult your veterinarian to learn which disorders are most common in your area.

Cervical Vertebral Myeloencephalopathy

For many years incoordinated horses were simply known as "wobblers." Today, the term refers primarily to horses with a developmental disorder of the cervical spine known as cervical vertebral myelopathy (CVM) or cervical stenotic myelopathy (CSM). The disease is common among young (one- to three-years-old), rapidly growing male horses of various breeds (Thoroughbreds, Standardbreds, large draft breeds). Narrowing of the spinal canal due to malformation of growing vertebrae and overriding adjacent vertebrae compresses the spinal cord. The cause of these developmental abnormalities appears to be related to genetic predisposition (conformation and growth potential) and diet (high carbohydrate, high zinc, low copper).

Proprioceptive tracts in the white matter are the most consistently and severely damaged, but motor pathways also can be affected. Although cord compression might occur in one or more sites, damage to the axons extends well above and below the local area of injury. The consistent nature of the damage is due to the relatively uniform nature of cord compression from the bottom and sides of the vertebral canal.

Affected horses exhibit characteristic clinical signs that primarily vary in degree of severity. These include symmetric ataxia and weakness (toe dragging, stumbling), which are usually worse in the rear legs. Clinical signs can become exaggerated by extending the neck up or bending it down. Infrequently, asymmetric ataxia can occur if degenerative vertebral joint disease (arthritis) becomes more severe on one side of the neck and compresses the spinal cord unilaterally. Neck pain is not usually associated with CVM; however, severe arthritic changes can result in bone growth that impinges on spinal nerves as they branch from the spinal cord and exit the spinal canal at vertebral joints. This results in neck pain, local muscle atrophy, and loss of cervical reflexes and skin sensation.

The diagnosis of CVM is greatly enhanced by the use of radiography (X-ray). Cervical radiographs taken with careful attention to detail provide a great deal of information regarding the likelihood of CVM. Unfortunately, many clinically normal horses have radiographic evidence of cervical vertebral joint disease. A more definitive diagnosis requires a myelogram. This is a series of special radiographs of the neck prepared by the addition of an X-ray-absorbing dye into the horse's spinal fluid. The dye is visible on radiographs of the spinal canal. Severe cord compression prevents the passage of dye through affected vetebral joint(s).

Nutritional and surgical therapies for CVM are available and have proven effective for many horses. However, improvement generally depends on the length of time clinical signs have been present prior to the initiation of treatment. This is simply a reflection of the poor regenerative ability of the CNS.

Trauma

Trauma is another common cause of neurologic deficits in the horse. Falls, collisions, kicks, and physical abuse can result in direct injury to nervous tissue with or without skull or vertebral fracture. Peripheral nerve damage is frequently associated with trauma and must be considered as well. Horses of all ages and breeds can be injured, but young, excitable horses and performance horses are more prone to accidental injury. The sudden onset of neurologic signs always suggests trauma, but it is important to remember that EPM can strike quickly and that horses with neurologic deficits are often predisposed to mishap. Fortunately, several factors help differentiate neurologic deficits due to traumatic injury from those associated with EPM.

Clinical signs depend on the location and severity of CNS injury. Horses might be down and comatose or simply appear stiff. Unlike with EPM, careful neurologic examination should localize damage to a single area of the CNS. Injuries to the brainstem and cervical spinal cord occur most frequently. Pain and external evidence of injury, such as swelling and skin damage, frequently are present at the site of impact. Radiographs often are helpful.

In the absence of displaced skull or vertebral fractures, initial trauma might result in minimal disruption of normal CNS architecture. However, hemorrhage and swelling within the bony confines of the CNS rapidly compromise the delivery of oxygen to neurons and other cells. Without rapid medical intervention, peak damage is usually reached within 24 hours. The clinical condition should then stablize or begin to improve without further progression, unless re-injury occurs. Depending on the severity of the injury, response to therapy can be rapid, very gradual over an extended period, or negligi-

UNDERSTANDING EPM

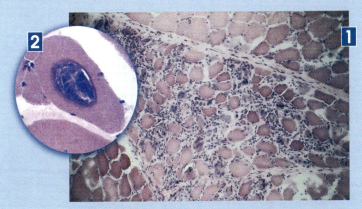

Inflammation and muscle degeneration caused by the *S. fayeri* sarcocyst, a species of *Sarcocystis*; inset: *S. fayeri* sarcocyst in the muscle.

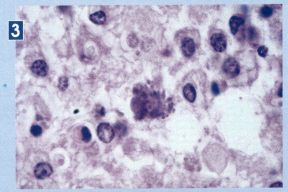

A section of spinal cord damaged by the EPM parasite.

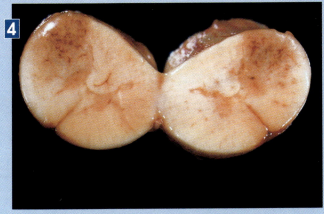

Spinal cord from an affected horse, showing hemorrhage and swelling.

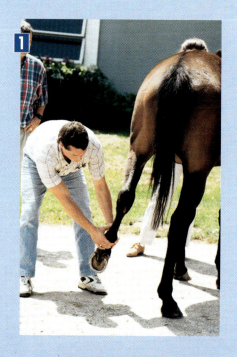

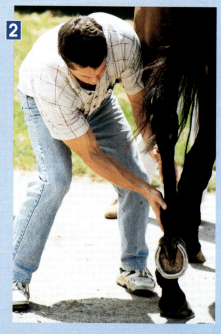

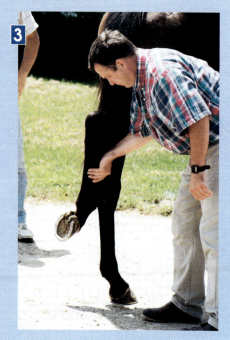

A thorough neurological exam is crucial in diagnosing EPM. In photos 1-3, the veterinarian assesses whether a horse knows where his rear limbs are placed. Many horses suffering from EPM experience a proprioceptive deficit, meaning their awareness of limb placement is compromised.

UNDERSTANDING EPM

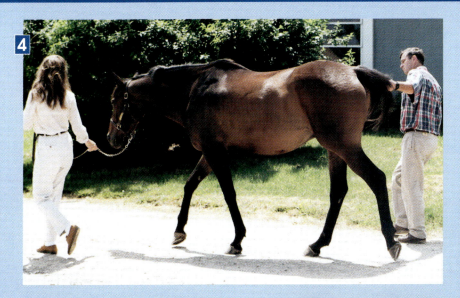

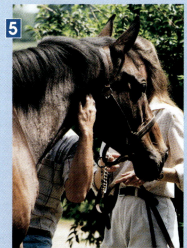

In photo 4, the veterinarian tests for weakness in the rear legs. In photo 5, the vet checks for assymetry in the muscles that are required for swallowing and the muscles that move the larynx. Below, the veterinarian draws cerebrospinal fluid for the EPM diagnostic test. The fluid can be drawn from the croup area or from behind the poll.

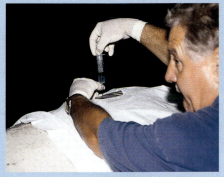

Lumbosacral CSF tap.

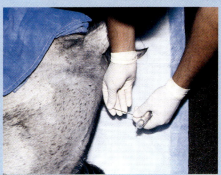

Atlanto-occipital CSF tap.

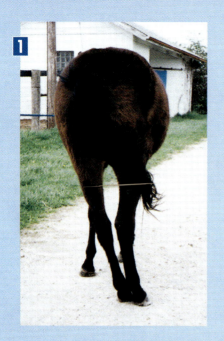
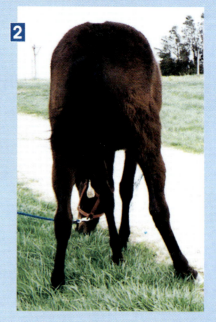
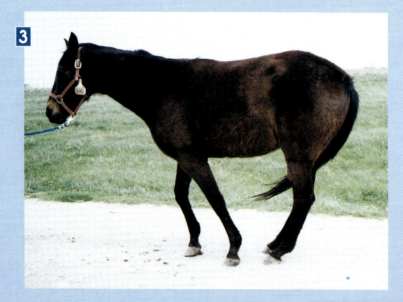

Rear limb incoordination, or ataxia, is perhaps the most common clinical sign of EPM. This horse is exhibiting abnormal body posture and placement of the rear legs.

UNDERSTANDING EPM

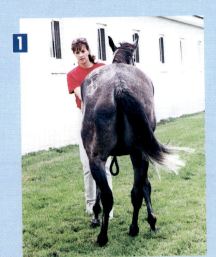

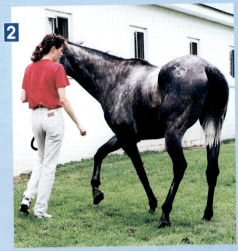

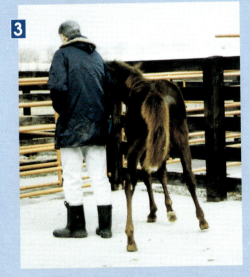

The horse in photos 1-2 has difficulty backing and knowing where his rear limbs are, both of which are signs associated with EPM.

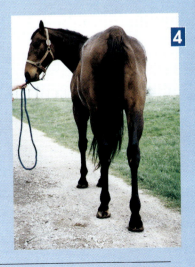

When turning, a horse with EPM frequently swings his outside rear leg out farther than normal, as does the horse in photo 3. The horse in photo 4 shows atrophy, or loss of muscle mass, another common sign of EPM.

53

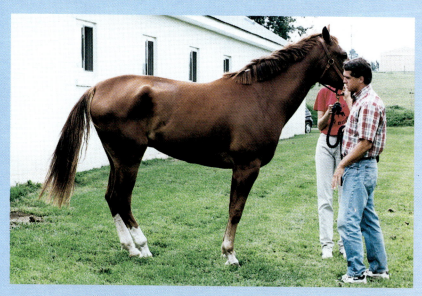

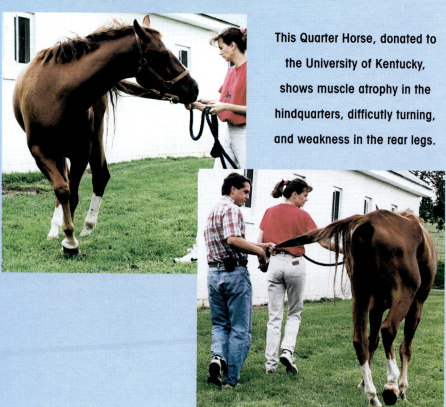

This Quarter Horse, donated to the University of Kentucky, shows muscle atrophy in the hindquarters, difficutly turning, and weakness in the rear legs.

UNDERSTANDING EPM

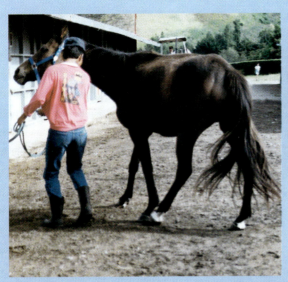
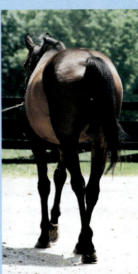

The clinical signs of EPM can vary from very abnormal body posture (top left) to mild ataxia (top right and bottom).

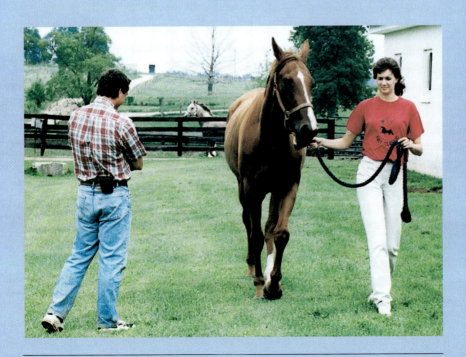

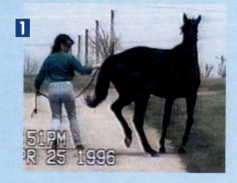
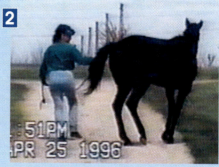
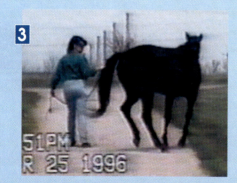
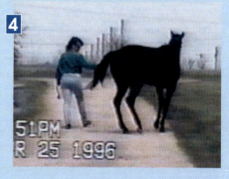
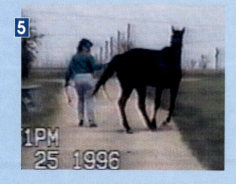

These photos were taken from a video of a mare with EPM before she began the experimental drug treatment program at the University of Kentucky. She now can walk straight and can fend for herself.

ble. Residual neurologic deficits are common.

Equine Degenerative Myeloencephalopathy

Equine degenerative myeloencephalopathy (EDM) is a very common neurologic disease of horses in the northeastern United States. It also occurs with somewhat less frequency in the rest of North America and Europe. The disease was first described in 1976 and, like EPM, it causes progressive ataxia and weakness in young horses of many breeds. Symmetric ataxia is common and generally most severe in the back legs. Clinical signs most often begin in weanlings and plateau by two years of age. Onset is usually insidious, although acute cases have been reported.

EDM has been linked to areas with limited pasture availability and reliance on pelleted feeds and hay. A great deal of evidence suggests that vitamin E deficiency and genetic predisposition are significant risk factors for EDM. Exposure to creosote wood preservatives and possibly pyrethrin insecticides might increase the risk of developing EDM. The disease produces diffuse, bilaterally symmetric degeneration of proprioceptive tracts in white matter of the spinal cord. Although lesions can develop in the brainstem, cranial nerve deficits do not occur. In addition, muscle atrophy and loss of skin sensation are not associated with EDM. If any of these signs develop, EDM can be dropped from the list of differential diagnoses. EDM is frequently diagnosed by a process of elimination as other neurologic diseases are removed from consideration by the results of diagnostic testing.

Affected horses are treated using daily, high-dose vitamin E supplementation for several years. Although some horses improve, EDM appears to be more effectively prevented than treated. Prevention also relies on daily vitamin E supplementation, but at a much lower dose.

Equine herpesvirus myeloencephalopathy

Equine herpesvirus-1 (EHV-1) is a contagious virus that causes abortion, upper respiratory, and neurologic disease among horses worldwide. The disease has produced outbreaks at breeding farms, training facilities, and racetracks. The virus has an affinity for vascular endothelial cells of the CNS, infecting them preferentially. Subsequent viral multiplication results in damage to the blood vessels (vasculitis), which interferes with oxygen delivery to the CNS. Gray and white matter of the spinal cord most often is affected, resulting in symmetric ataxia and weakness of the rear legs, bladder paralysis, and loss of tail and anal tone. Treatment often is successful if affected horses retain the ability to stand. Some recover rapidly while others improve gradually for many months. Residual neurologic deficits may remain. EHV-1 vaccines are available, but have been unable to prevent neurologic disease.

OTHER NEUROLOGIC DISEASES

EPM, trauma, CVM, and EDM account for the vast majority of equine neurologic diseases in North America. However, a number of other neurologic diseases that are easily confused with EPM occur sporadically.

Otitis Media/Interna

Middle and inner ear infection (otitis media/interna) and temporohyoid osteoarthropathy involve progressive inflammation of the middle ear and the associated joint between the temporal and stylohyoid bones. The underlying cause of middle ear disease is believed to be chronic middle ear infection that spreads to the bone. Chronic arthritis of the temporohyoid joint results in fusion of the joint and loss of normal mobility. Pressure develops from movement of the tongue and larynx, resulting in fracture of the the skull and occasionally the stylohyoid bone. Initially, horses exhibit signs of ear pain, such as ear rubbing, head tossing, and sensitivity to touch.

Continued arthritic changes damage cranial nerve VII (facial) and VIII (vestibulocochlear), resulting in facial paralysis, head tilt, and ataxia.

Occasionally, cranial nerves IX (glossopharyngeal) and X (vagus) are injured as well, resulting in difficulty eating and swallowing (dysphagia).

Blindfolding horses with ataxia due to vestibulocochlear nerve or associated brainstem damage will make them unable to compensate visually for the loss of balance and make the ataxia much worse. Radiographs and video endoscope examination of the guttural pouches are also helpful. Antibacterial and anti-inflammatory therapy, as well as surgical intervention, has proven to be effective therapies that frequently return horses to normal function.

Verminous Encephalomyelitis

Various parasites (worms and fly larvae) inadvertently migrate into the CNS during part of their developmental cycle. Several are primary equine parasites, some are misplaced from other animals, and still others are free-living opportunists. Most worms gain entry through ingestion and penetration of the gut to reach the bloodstream. One type enters the bloodstream through mosquito bites, while the most common type (*Halicephalobus deletrix*) enters the nose while horses are drinking. Heel fly larvae penetrate the skin and migrate directly to the CNS.

Fortunately, parasite migration in the CNS is rare. Clinical signs are variable and depend on the route of migration. Asymmetric, multifocal signs are most common. The brain is affected more frequently than the spinal cord. Onset is typically sudden, and the course of infection is usually rapid. However, chronic infections have been reported. Differential diagnosis is difficult. Occasionally, microscopic evaluation of CSF reveals a white blood cell type (eosinophil) that is associated with the presence of worms. Treatment includes anti-inflammatory drugs, antiparasitic drugs, and good nursing care. Although residual neurologic deficits are common, many horses respond favorably to treatment.

Cauda Equina Syndrome

Cauda equina syndrome refers to a set of neurologic deficits that result from damage to the sacral spinal cord and its spinal nerves. *Cauda equina* literally means "horse tail" in Latin and refers to the physical resemblance of the many branching spinal nerves to a horse's tail. The clinical signs of cauda equina syndrome are identical to those described for EHV-1. In fact, EHV-1, as well as EPM, trauma, tumors, abcesses, migrating parasites (worms), and ingestion of sorghum-sudan grass are all considered causes of cauda equina syndrome. Polyneuritis equi is a very similar syndrome which affects older horses and is believed to be caused by a misdirected immune response against the horse's own CNS. Progressive inflammation of the sacral spinal cord and brainstem can occur. Cranial nerve signs include facial paralysis, jaw muscle atrophy, head tilt, and loss of equilibrium with ataxia. Successful treatment of cauda equina syndrome is dependent on the underlying cause. Treatment of polyneuritis equi is unrewarding.

Rabies

Although rabies virus infection is relatively uncommon in the horse, it should always be considered when neurologic deficits have been present for less than 10 days. Rabies usually results in death in three to 10 days unless anti-inflammatory drugs prolong the course inadvertently. Clinical signs of rabies are highly variable and can include ataxia, rear limb weakness, extremely sensitive skin, and atypical or aggressive behavior. The disease inevitably progresses to coma and death unless it is recognized quickly and the horse euthanized. The disease can be effectively prevented with the use of available vaccines.

Neoplasia

Benign or malignant tumors of the CNS and associated tissues are relatively uncommon but do occur. Clinical signs are directly related to compression of the affected area and typically are asymmetric and progressive. Lymphosarcomas are probably the most frequently diagnosed tumors in the CNS. They usually are spread throughout the rest of the body as well. Thorough examination might reveal more superficial tumors and enlarged lymph nodes, which will aid in the diagnosis. Radiographs and myelograms can help differentiate some tumors. Horses usually do not respond to treatment.

Many neurologic disorders that have not been discussed occur in horses. Hopefully, most will agree that those left out are either easily differentiated from EPM or occur too infrequently in most of North America for consideration here. These disorders include other viral, bacterial, and fungal CNS infections; bacterial vertebral infection; epidural abcesses; tetanus; botulism; mycotoxins (moldy corn poisoning); Lyme disease; toxic plants or chemicals; metabolic disorders (liver disease, hypoglycemia); congenital abnormalities; motor neuron disease; postanesthetic hemorrhagic myelopathy; epilepsy; and narcolepsy. Consult your veterinarian if you need additional information regarding any of these disorders.

ANCILLARY DIAGNOSTIC AIDS

The usefulness of nerve blocks, radiographs, myelograms, and video endoscopy has been discussed. Other useful diagnostic aids include nuclear scintigraphy, electromyograms (EMG), electroencephalograms (EEG), ultrasound, thermography, computed tomography (CT scan), and magnetic resonance imaging (MRI). Many of these techniques are available only at large referral centers and veterinary teaching hospitals. Although very few veterinarians have access to CT and MRI, these technologies have proven to be extremely helpful for the diagnosis of equine neurologic diseases. Hopefully, they will become more widely available in the future.

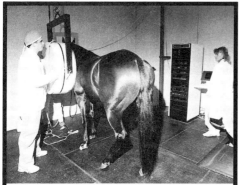
Scintigraphy can be a useful aid in diagnosing neurological diseases.

LABORATORY TESTING

Laboratory diagnostic tests provide a useful adjunct to clincal examination for the differentiation of EPM from other neurologic diseases. A number of laboratory tests are available. Complete (CBC) and differential blood counts help differentiate various types of infectious and non-infectious diseases by evaluation of the number, type, and characteristics of red and white blood cells present in a blood sample. Veterinarians often evaluate multiple blood samples over a period of days or weeks to monitor changes that might suggest a diagnosis or indicate a change in the condition. Unfortunately, EPM rarely causes any detectable changes in the CBC or differential cell count.

Serum chemistry profiles include a broad array of tests to evaluate electrolyte balance, hydration, liver and kidney function, muscle damage, inflammatory activity, and antibody production. Although these tests can help diagnose other diseases, EPM does not produce any consistent changes.

Muscle samples can be collected and processed to differentiate primary muscle disorders from loss of innervation. EMGs also are used to evaluate muscle innervation.

Cerebrospinal fluid (CSF) samples can be collected and analyzed for a number of factors that often are useful for differentiation between infectious and non-infectious neurologic diseases. These include color, clarity, cell counts, and concentration of protein, enzymes, glucose, electrolytes, and antibody. Blood contamination of CSF during the spinal tap and sample collection is common and, unfortunately, precludes useful analysis of the sample. When this occurs, the horse should be re-tapped in a few days. This does not appear to jeopardize the reliability of test results. It should be remembered that traumatic injury and verminous encephalomyelitis also can cause hemorrhage into the CSF. Nonetheless, EPM rarely produces consistent changes in these parameters.

The ratio of CSF protein (albumin) concentration to serum albumin concentration provides an index called the albumin quotient (AQ). Albumin is the major protein of serum and is not produced in CSF. It must enter the CSF from serum. Therefore, comparing AQ from abnormal horses to the range of values for AQ established from normal horses helps veterinarians determine the integrity of the blood-brain barrier. If the CSF albumin concentration is significantly elevated, accidental blood contamination of the sample must be considered.

> **AT A GLANCE**
>
> - Various laboratory tests can help distinguish EPM from other neurological diseases.
>
> - The presence of antibodies to the EPM parasite in blood and cerebrospinal fluid is the basis of the EPM diagnostic test.
>
> - One study found that testing cerebrospinal fluid would detect *S. neurona* antibodies in nine out of 10 horses showing neurological signs of EPM.
>
> - Immunoblot and DNA testing can help determine exposure to *S. neurona*.

Immunoglobulin type G (IgG) is the most abundant class of antibody produced in the horse. Total IgG concentration is determined in CSF and serum, and the ratio is used in conjunction with the AQ to evaluate local IgG production in the CNS. EPM, as well as some other CNS diseases, routinely causes elevated IgG production in the CNS.

The presence of the *S. neurona*-specific antibody in serum and CSF is the basis of the EPM diagnostic test. The EPM test was developed in 1991 using cultured *S. neurona* merozoites and antiserum from horses with EPM or *S. fayeri* exposure. Rabbit antisera against *S. neurona*, *S. cruzi*, and *S. muris* also were used for comparison. Cultured merozoites were dissolved and individual proteins in the mixture were electrically separated in a thin sheet of clear gel (electrophoresis). A piece of paper was placed over the gel, and an electric current was used to transfer (blot) the separated proteins onto the paper. This made it possible to compare the reactivity of antibodies produced against several *Sarcocystis* to *S. neurona* proteins (immunoblot analysis).

Eight unique proteins that reacted only with antibodies produced against *S. neurona* were identified. Several of these proteins became the basis of the EPM test developed at the University of Kentucky, then transferred to the university-owned Equine Biodiagnostics, Inc. in 1995.

Although we have continued to make improvements in the EPM test over the years, it still is based on the original immunoblot technique. Every aspect of the test has been optimized and standardized for maximum sensitivity and specificity, as well as minimal test-to-test variation. Extensive internal and external control samples are run on every blot to ensure the accuracy and reliability of each result.

A fluorescent immunoassay (FIAX) based on *S. cruzi* bradyzoites isolated from cattle muscle has been available to test horses for *Sarcocystis* exposure since the mid-1980s. The test relies on antibodies in equine serum that cross-react with *S. cruzi* proteins. This means that many non-specific antibodies to *S. fayeri* and *S. neurona* present in a horse's serum will react in the test. Since approximately 30% of horses are believed to be exposed to *S. fayeri*, the usefulness of this test is questionable. Shared serum samples have demonstrated that those with positive FIAX values might test negative by immunoblot analysis. Similarly, sera with negative FIAX values have tested positve on immunoblot. The FIAX test is attractive to veterinarians because it provides an approximate numerical measure of the amount of antibody present. Veterinarians like to know if serum antibody concentration is increasing or decreasing over time to determine if an infection is recent or on its way out. However, EPM confounds the use of antibody concentration whether FIAX values are accurate or not.

Horses with active EPM might have extremely low amounts of serum (or CSF) antibody. Occasionally, affected horses have even tested negative. If *any* specific antibody is detected in the serum (or CSF), the horse has been exposed. The parasite has proven its ability to cause disease months after initial exposure. Presumably, serum antibodies rise following each exposure and begin to fall shortly after the parasite crosses the blood-brain barrier and enters the CNS. An exposure rate of 45% indicates that horses probably ingest sporocysts on a fairly routine basis. Therefore, it makes little difference if serum (or CSF) antibody concentration is high or low or if it is going up or down; it only matters whether antibodies are present or not, that is, if the sample tests positive or negative.

Immunoblot testing of equine serum and CSF provides veterinarians with valuable information regarding exposure to *S. neurona*. Antibodies directed against proteins shared by *S. fayeri* and similar organisms are differentiated. A recent report based on data from a horse which had died due to *Neospora caninum* encephalitis suggested that antibodies produced against *N. caninum* cross-react with some *S. neurona*-specific proteins. However, careful evaluation of the material presented indicates that the information was confounded. The horse clearly was exposed to *S. neurona*, as well as *N. caninum*. Presumably, anti-*S. neurona* antibodies from serum were present in CSF. Alternatively, *S. neurona* merozoites also were present in the CNS. A controlled experimental infection study done in an isolation facility using horses with no anti-protozoal antibodies in serum or CSF would be required to evaluate this hypothesis accurately. A related study, using rabbit antiserum prepared against *S. neurona* and *N. caninum*, failed to demonstrate any cross-reactivity with the specific proteins.

The results of EPM tests on CSF samples from 295 horses euthanized due to neurologic disease were compared to postmortem diagnoses. Many equine neurologic diseases were represented in the study. Approximately 40% of the horses had postmortem diagnoses of EPM. The sensitivity and specificity of CSF test results were both approximately 90%. Sensitivity reflects the number of horses that tested CSF positive out of all horses diagnosed with EPM at postmortem. Specificity reflects the number of horses that tested CSF negative from all the horses that did not have EPM at postmortem. These results indicate that the EPM test would detect *S. neurona* antibodies in the CSF of nine out of 10 horses showing neurologic signs. Several of the horses which tested false negative had been ill for less than three weeks.

Although the incubation period of EPM appears to be sufficient to permit production of detectable amounts of specific antibody in most cases, false negative CSF test results do occur. It is advisable to re-test horses with acute neurologic disease which initially test negative. Nonetheless, some horses remain negative and simply fail to produce a detectable antibody response to the specific proteins used for analysis.

Specificity of 90% suggests that one in 10 horses with neurologic signs would test positive for *S. neurona* antibodies in CSF even though they have another neurologic disease. Whenever the integrity of the blood-brain barrier is compromised, antibodies from the blood stream can leak into the CSF and produce a false positive test result. False positive CSF test results were noted from cases of CVM, viral encephalitis, trauma, EDM, moldy corn poisoning, and CNS abcess. However, the most common cause of false positive test results for CSF is blood contamination at the time of collection. The AQ, total albumin, and red blood cell count should help determine if CSF has been blood contaminated or the blood-brain barrier has been damaged.

It is very important to note that sensitivity and specificity were calculated using CSF from horses which had obvious neurologic disease. They should not be extrapolated to interpret CSF test results for horses without neurologic signs. As discussed previously, not enough is known about the activity of *S. neurona* in the horse for adequate interpretation of CSF test results from normal horses. Understandably, it is disconcerting to realize that parasites are likely to be present in the CNS whenever antibodies are detected in CSF; nonetheless, the likelihood of clinical disease is unknown.

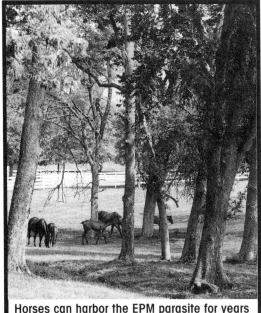

Horses can harbor the EPM parasite for years without exhibiting signs of disease.

The horse might become ill tomorrow, two years from now, or not at all. Opinions on how to handle this situation differ widely. It seems reasonable to assume that the horse is handling the parasite adequately for the moment, but how will the battle go tomorrow? Since we do not know the likelihood of complete parasite elimination without treatment, but can easily appreciate how quickly the disease can cause permanent damage, a single round (three to four months) of standard therapy seems reasonable.

Many excellent veterinarians disagree with this approach. Their concern might be justified. Treatment is expensive and not without some risk. It is entirely possible that we eventually will discover that the vast majority of these horses actually eliminate the parasite without treatment. It should be clear that, for the moment, CSF test results from normal horses cannot be adequately interpreted to justify consideration during the sale of a horse.

Seroprevalence studies of normal horse populations have shown that a positive EPM blood test result indicates exposure only. The relatively few number of EPM cases compared to the large number of exposed horses suggests that many are exposed, but few become ill. The sensitivity and specificity of EPM *blood* test results from the 295 horse postmortem study reinforce these findings. Sensitivity was approximately 90%, but specificity was only 70%. Most of the horses with EPM tested positive, but 30% of those with other neurologic disease did as well. The real value of EPM blood testing among normal horses appears to be a negative test.

Parasite DNA-specific polymerase chain reaction (PCR) testing of CSF also provides information regarding the presence of *S. neurona* in the CNS. Although the sensitivity of PCR testing is apparently much lower than initially estimated, the demonstrated ability to detect parasite DNA in false negative CSF samples makes it a useful adjunct for the diagnosis of EPM in selected cases. Parasite DNA can be rapidly destroyed by enzymatic action in the CSF and appears to find its way into the CSF rarely during the course of infection.

RESEARCH IN PROGRESS: NEW AND IMPROVED TESTS

Specific diagnostic methods for EPM have advanced significantly the last few years. However, further enhancement of current methods and the development of alternate technologies are needed. Various laboratories around the United States are working on commercial diagnostic tests for EPM using various formats, including immunoblot, enzyme linked immunosorbant assays (ELISA), and PCR. Understanding the last part of the parasite life cycle and identification of various parasite strains should occur soon and will assist in the development of highly specific target antigen preparations for immunologic testing.

The development of accurate diagnostic tests for other equine neurologic diseases will help differentiate these diseases from EPM more efficiently. PCR assays for several viral CNS diseases are currently used on a research basis, but are not yet commercially available.

Case Review I

The following case review illustrates many of the points discussed and provides a typical example of the case histories used to develop the recommendations found in this text

A 7-year-old Thoroughbred mare began dragging her right rear toe and seemed slightly lame. The mare was bright and alert, but had difficulty eating and dropped a large amount of sweet feed each day. Her condition gradually worsened over the next two weeks, and she began to stumble when ridden. The mare was a lightly used pleasure horse.

The owner consulted a veterinarian

Vaccinations and de-worming had been done on a regular schedule and were up to date. The mare had not been ill or injured in the last year. The owner had taken her on a trail ride in a neighboring county four weeks earlier. Temperature, pulse, and respiratory rate were normal.

A neurologic exam revealed abnormal tongue strength and loss of tail tone as well as delayed placing reactions and ataxia involving the rear limbs. This condition was more pronounced on the left. Based on the presence of progressive multifocal neurologic signs and the age of the horse, the veterinarian discounted the possibility of cervical vertebral myeloencephalopathy, trauma, or equine degenerative myeloencephalopathy. The clinical signs and history suggested EPM, but equine herpes myeloencephalopathy and cauda equina/polyneuritis equi remained possibilities.

An inspection of the barn revealed a family of opossums living in the hay loft. The veterinarian decided to place the mare on standard therapy for EPM and attempted to confirm the diagnosis by testing serum and cerebrospinal fluid for the presence of *S. neurona*-specific antibodies.

Routine blood work, including CBC, differential cell count, and serum chemistries, was normal. Serum and CSF both tested positive in the EPM test. CSF was clear and colorless. CSF albumin, AQ, IgG index, and cell counts were within normal limits. In addition, the mare was responding to treatment. She appeared to recover fully after three months and treatment was discontinued.

Relapse, then progress

Six weeks later she began dragging her right rear toe and dropping grain. The owner immediately called the veterinarian, and the mare was started on standard therapy. Her condition failed to improve. After three months, the mare was still dragging her toe. Blood and spinal fluid samples were taken, and both tested positive in the EPM test. The mare was placed on a double dose of standard therapy. Clinical signs slowly improved and appeared to stabilize after three months. Although the blood test was still positive, CSF tested negative. Treatment was discontinued, and the mare did not relapse in subsequent months.

Case Review II

A two-year-old Thoroughbred gelding began training poorly. Neurologic examination revealed mild asymmetric ataxia of the rear limbs. A presumptive diagnosis of EPM was made, and the horse was placed on standard therapy. An EPM blood test was positive. Gradual improvement was noted, and training was resumed. Treatment was discontinued after three months, but clinical signs returned within four weeks.

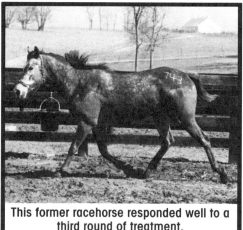

This former racehorse responded well to a third round of treatment.

The horse was placed on treatment again and responded gradually. Training was resumed, and the horse was raced several months later while still on treatment. The horse performed poorly, and mild ataxia was still present. The horse was removed from training and rested for several weeks without treatment. Clinical signs became progressively worse. EPM tests on both blood and spinal fluid were positive.

Deterioration, then improvement

Treatment was started, and the horse dramatically worsened and was unable to stand. The condition did not respond rapidly to anti-inflammatory drugs, and the horse was placed in a sling. Gradual improvement was noted, and the sling was removed after eight weeks.

Treatment was discontinued, and the horse was turned out daily into increasingly larger paddocks to exercise until he was able to return to pasture. The horse has slight residual neurologic deficits but has not relapsed after eight months.

NEUROLOGICAL EXAMINATION FORM

Horse Name/I.D. _____

Breed: _____ Sex: _____ Body Weight: _____

Date of Examination: _____

1) **Appetite:**

Food Consumption:	Normal	Abnormal
Water Consumption:	Normal	Abnormal

2) **Attitude/Behavior**

Anxious	No	Yes
Apprehensive	No	Yes
Convulsions	No	Yes
Depressed	No	Yes
Head Pressing	No	Yes
Nose or lip wrinkled	No	Yes
Shaking Head	No	Yes
Tongue Hanging Out	No	Yes

3) **Head Evaluation**

Tilt	No	Yes
Symmetry	No	Yes
Lip droop/salivation	No	Yes
Intention Tremor	No	Yes
Sensation	No	Yes
Swallow (gag)	No	Yes
Tongue Tone	No	Yes

Other:

Cranial Nerves	Left		Right	
Vision	Normal	Abnormal	Normal	Abnormal
Pupil size/symmetry	Normal	Abnormal	Normal	Abnormal
Pupillary light reflex	Normal	Abnormal	Normal	Abnormal
Menace Response	Normal	Abnormal	Normal	Abnormal
Blink to bright light	Normal	Abnormal	Normal	Abnormal
Corneal Reflex	Normal	Abnormal	Normal	Abnormal
Strabismus	Normal	Abnormal	Normal	Abnormal
Nystagmus	Normal	Abnormal	Normal	Abnormal
Facial Muscle Tone	Normal	Abnormal	Normal	Abnormal
Mastication muscle tone	Normal	Abnormal	Normal	Abnormal

4) **Body Evaluation**

Body Sensation	Left		Right	
Neck	Normal	Abnormal	Normal	Abnormal
Trunk	Normal	Abnormal	Normal	Abnormal
Limbs	Normal	Abnormal	Normal	Abnormal
Quarter	Normal	Abnormal	Normal	Abnormal
Perianal	Normal	Abnormal	Normal	Abnormal

Muscle Atrophy	Left		Right	
Neck	Normal	Abnormal	Normal	Abnormal
Back	Normal	Abnormal	Normal	Abnormal
Limbs	Normal	Abnormal	Normal	Abnormal
Quarter	Normal	Abnormal	Normal	Abnormal
Tail	Normal	Abnormal	Normal	Abnormal

Other:

5) Gait Evaluation

Gait Symmetry (describe): _____ Walking: _____ Head Raised: _____

	Walking			Head Raised		
Truncal Swaying	No	Yes	Worsens	No	Yes	Worsens
Toe dragging (If yes, which limb:) _____	No	Yes	Worsens	No	Yes	Worsens
Inconsistent Limb Placement (If yes, which limb:) _____	No	Yes	Worsens	No	Yes	Worsens
Limb Interference (If yes, which limb:) _____	No	Yes	Worsens	No	Yes	Worsens
Pacing	No	Yes	Worsens	No	Yes	Worsens

Circling left: Circumduction RR limb   No   Yes _____

Toe dragging   No   Yes   (If yes, which limb: _____)

Other:

Circling right Circumduction LR limb   No   Yes

Toe dragging   No   Yes   If yes, which limb: _____)

Other:

Placing Reactions	Left		Right	
Front	Normal	Abnormal	Normal	Abnormal
Rear	Normal	Abnormal	Normal	Abnormal

Hoofwear:

Front	Normal Abnormal	Normal Abnormal
Rear	Normal Abnormal	Normal Abnormal

Backing:

Toe dragging	No	Yes
Pacing	No	Yes
Inconsistent Placement	No	Yes

Grade Scale for Ataxia, Weakness, & Spasticity: 1 to 5 (5 being the worst)

Ataxia: _____ Spasticity: _____ Weakness: _____

CHAPTER 4
How EPM is Treated?

Use of the term "standard therapy" is somewhat misleading. Different treatment protocols are in current use. Each veterinarian develops preferences based on personal experience. However, the essential elements of effective therapy include the use of pyrimethamine (Daraprim) and a sulfa drug. The drugs act in sequence to interfere with the parasite's ability to produce an essential requirement for DNA replication. In sufficient amounts, the combination acts synergistically to prevent parasite multiplication. Although the drugs are unable to kill parasites directly, they do slow them down enough to allow the horse's immune response to gain control.

For many years, veterinary texts recommended the use of a sulfa drug — trimethoprim combination (sulfadiazine in Tribrissen or sulfamethoxazole in SMZ-TMP) with pyrimethamine. The need for trimethoprim was questioned when it was realized that the dose used to treat EPM (15-30 mg/kg as a combined dose twice daily) would result in CSF concentrations below the amount necessary to inhibit similar protozoa in laboratory tests. Since the inclusion of trimethoprim also increased the likelihood of anemia and diarrhea, many dropped it from their recommendations. However, some veterinarians believe that horses respond faster and have fewer relapses when trimethoprim is included with standard therapy. Studies of past and future cases conducted at large veterinary referral centers and veterinary teaching hospitals should help resolve this issue.

Early pyrimethamine recommendations (0.25 mg/kg once daily for 30 days) appear to have been inadequate. Experience and a 1992 study demonstrating pyrimethamine's relatively poor ability to cross the blood-brain barrier prompted a dramatic increase in the amount of pyrimethamine recommended (0.5-1.0 mg/kg once daily) for treatment.

In addition, the frequent lack of rapid improvement and post-treatment relapse led to an increase in the length of treatment (eight weeks). It quickly was recognized that the variability of response to treatment was too great to rely on a set length of treatment. The current recommendation — to continue treatment for a least one month after the horse stops showing further improvement — has become generally accepted over the last few years. Using this rule of thumb, the average length of treatment approaches four months.

VARYING RESULTS WITH STANDARD TREATMENT

The most common form of treatment now recommended uses a commercially prepared liquid formulation of sulfadiazine and pyrimethamine, which delivers 20 mg/kg sulfadiazine and 1.0 mg/kg pyrimethamine at the recommended dose once daily. This appears to work reasonably well, but initial treatment failure or relapse still occurs. Referral centers using this protocol have reported up to a 75% response rate, although less than 25% of these made a full recovery. Mildly affected horses treated early in the course of infection have a much greater opportunity for complete recovery. Chronic signs of CNS damage such as muscle atrophy rarely improve. Some veterinarians recommend a second daily dose of sulfadiazine. It is not clear if this has an appreciable effect on the response to therapy.

Relapse following treatment continues to be a problem. It has been estimated that neurologic signs return within a few weeks or months of therapy in 10% to 25% of horses treated according to current recommendations. Many veterinarians have attempted to reduce the number of relapses by continuing treatment until the EPM test on CSF is negative. In theory, parasite-specific antibodies should clear the CSF within a few weeks of parasite elimination. Experience suggests that an extremely low number of horses relapse when CSF is negative at the time treatment is discontinued. The majority of horses should test CSF negative by the time the rule of thumb for treatment length has been fully applied.

However, it has become apparent that some horses remain CSF positive for an extended period after full recovery or stabilization without further improvement. The most likely explanation for this is the continued presence of parasites in the CNS. Some veterinarians theorize that the parasites have been eliminated and that the test remains positive due to antibody leakage from the bloodstream and/or an unknown mechanism that causes continued antibody production in the CNS without the presence of parasites. Although leakage is certainly responsible in some cases, there have been too many with normal total albumin, AQ, and an elevated IgG index for this to be responsible. Not all horses taken off treatment with positive CSF relapse. Some could have eliminated the parasite recently, and some will eliminate the parasite on their own. Certainly, it is very cumbersome, expensive, and usually impractical to treat horses indefinitely.

FINDING THE RIGHT DOSAGE

At some point it becomes necessary to question the adequacy of the recommended dosage. In other words, if the failure or relapse rates are unacceptable, is it more reasonable to increase the drug dose or to continue extending the length of treatment? Increasing the dosage does increase the potential for more severe side effects. These include anemia, low white blood cell counts, and short-term depression. Some researchers also have suggested that abortion and decreased stallion fertility might occur; however, controlled studies to prove these theories have not been done in the horse. It seems most reasonable to increase the dose within safe limits and to maintain the rule of thumb regarding the length of treatment. Many veterinarians are now recommending 1.5 to two times the dose of pyrimethamine for initial treatment or after 30 days if there is not satisfactory progress.

An increase in side effects has not been a problem to date. However, a monthly complete blood count is recommended to monitor anemia when using standard therapy and would be even more important at the higher dose. Some veterinarians also monitor serum folate concentration at monthly intervals. It is advisable to avoid higher doses in pregnant mares until more is known about the effects of therapy. Hopefully this will shorten the length of time required for treatment and reduce the number of horses that persistently test positive in CSF.

When relapse does occur, it is important to double the dose of pyrimethamine during the re-treatment. Unless the horse has become re-infected (which might be extremely unusual), the population of parasites causing the problem are directly descended from those most resistant to the first round of therapy. It is unreasonable to assume that use of the same dose would accomplish much more than another relapse.

> **AT A GLANCE**
>
> - The use of pyrimethamine (Daraprim) and a sulfa drug are the essential elements of effective therapy.
>
> - The two drugs used together can prevent the parasite from multiplying, but cannot kill it.
>
> - Most horses respond to the standard therapy, but less than one-quarter make a full recovery.
>
> - Relapses are common.
>
> - Horses attempting to recover from EPM should not be placed in stressful situations.
>
> - The University of Kentucky has reported success treating EPM horses with the experimental drug diclazuril.

Medication or supplements to stimulate the immune system might help, but no reports of improved treatment response have been published. It is possible that they could even exacerbate problems by increasing the amount of CNS inflammation.

When a double dose of pyrimethamine has been used for three to four months following relapse and the CSF continues to test positive, few choices remain. These would include indefinite treatment, an even higher pyrimethamine dosage, discontinuation of treatment and close monitoring, or use of an experimental drug. Experimental drugs are experimental for a reason. They may not work and they might be toxic. Do not even consider use of an experimental drug until all standard therapeutic options have been exhausted.

GIVE MEDICATION PROPERLY

Appropriate delivery of the medication can make a significant difference in the outcome of treatment. The sulfa-pyrimethamine liquid should be given on an empty stomach to prevent interference with absorption from the gut. Grass and hay have been shown to decrease the uptake of these drugs. Feed should be withheld for at least two hours before and one hour after administration. Although grain causes much less interference than grass and hay, it is still far better to place the medication directly in the horse's mouth than on the feed. Horses which do not receive an adequate amount of the drugs will not improve. In fact, erratic blood concentrations that dip below the amount required to impair parasite division will encourage the development of drug-resistant strains. Your time, effort, money, and horse will be wasted.

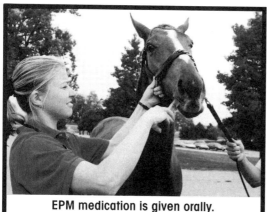
EPM medication is given orally.

Anti-inflammatory drugs during the first one to two weeks of treatment and any time the condition appears to worsen during treatment should help minimize further damage due to parasite death and the host response. Dimethyl sulfoxide (DMSO) and flunixin meglumine (Banamine) or phenylbutazone are used most frequently. Horses which are severely affected often receive moderate doses of dexamethasone for one to three days. Longer use might cause suppression of the immune response. Oral vitamin E supplementation (10-20 international units/kg daily) also is recommended to promote healing of the CNS.

Recently, it was noted that folic acid is poorly absorbed by horses. Therefore, folic acid supplementation for prevention or treatment of anemia and prevention of potential pregnancy problems during standard EPM therapy is not likely to be effective. Folinic acid (a variant of folic acid) is well absorbed and highly effective in other species, but the cost of supplemental administration in the horse is prohibitive. Fortunately, good quality pasture and alfalfa hay are an excellent source of folinic acid and are highly recommended during treatment. If life-threatening anemia develops, your veterinarian either will have to try folinic acid therapy or discontinue treatment for two to three weeks to allow recovery.

AVOID STRESS DURING RECOVERY

It is important not to stress horses attempting to recover from EPM. The amount of activity appropriate for each case is highly variable and dependent on the circumstances surrounding the individual. Horses which are severely affected should be confined in a heavily bedded box stall

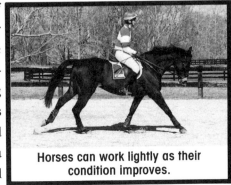
Horses can work lightly as their condition improves.

until they are able to move easily. Try to avoid making any dramatic changes in the horse's environment to avoid stress. Prolonged inactivity is not beneficial. Light exercise is appropriate as improvement of the condition permits. Work can be increased gradually as the horse improves and drug therapy nears completion. It is better to be patient and to avoid overworking a horse on treatment. At best, too much work too soon prolongs the length of time to full recovery and the return to normal activity. At worst, there will be an opportunity for a postmortem diagnosis.

ALTERNATIVE THERAPY

Chiropractic, massage therapy, and acupuncture all seem to help sore horses feel better. Because asymmetric ataxia can produce soreness and injury, these therapies should be helpful. None of these methods eliminate parasites by themselves, but they can serve as a useful adjunct to standard therapy. This is not an endorsement for diagnosis of EPM using

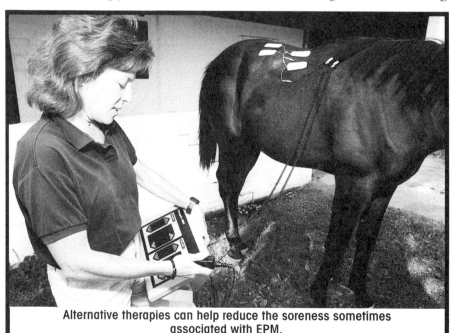

Alternative therapies can help reduce the soreness sometimes associated with EPM.

acupuncture. The accuracy of this technique has not been substantiated experimentally.

RESEARCH IN PROGRESS: NEW DRUGS

Work on the triazine antiprotozoal drug group is being done at the University of Kentucky. This drug group is attractive because it is generally safe for use in mammals and is able to kill protozoa in laboratory tests instead of simply preventing their multiplication. No member of the group has been approved for use in the United States. The University of Kentucky has an investigational new animal drug permit from the Federal Drug Administration to import the drug, diclazuril, for experimental use. The preliminary study is in the final stages.

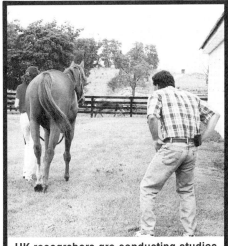

UK researchers are conducting studies with an experimental drug.

Very strict clinical criteria have been established to satisfy the requirements necessary for FDA approval of new animal drugs in phase II of this study. It is necessary to screen all horses carefully for entry into these trials. A small percentage of affected horses will be eligible.

Efficacy and toxicity trials are planned.

Diclazuril has been used to treat a number of severely affected horses successfully. While we remain optimistic, not all results have been favorable. There is no guarantee that diclazuril or other triazines will be superior to standard therapy. Hopefully, the drug will at least provide another choice when resistance develops to standard therapy. It also might prove to be useful in combination with standard therapy to enhance performance and prevent resistance.

CHAPTER 5

How can EPM be Prevented?

Horse owners and managers can take a number of positive steps to help reduce the risk of EPM for the horses in their care. Prevention can be broken down into three basic areas: health and condition, facility maintenance, and travel planning.

HEALTH & CONDITION

A healthy, fit horse is the best protection you can have for the prevention of many equine diseases, and EPM is no exception. As we have discussed, the horse's immune system is the key to overcoming EPM. The development of clinical signs appears to be related to the number of sporocysts ingested, but the ability of an individual to resist infection will affect the actual number of sporocysts required. Therefore, all of the routine preventive health care recommendations apply to EPM as well. These include routine vaccinations, regular de-worming, proper nutri-

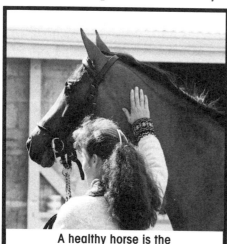
A healthy horse is the best defense.

tion, plenty of exercise, routine foot care, preventive dental care, and routine examination by your veterinarian. Performance horses should be properly conditioned to avoid injury and overwork. Small health problems can lead quickly to large ones when ignored. The stress associated with other diseases might provide an ideal opportunity for *S. neurona* to emerge from hiding.

Horses experience mental as well as physical stress. Careful attention to the personality and individual needs of each horse will reduce stress. Whenever possible, avoid unnecessary management decisions that will introduce significant changes in the horse's physical and social environment. This is especially important when other stressful events are scheduled.

It is very important to seek prompt veterinary assistance whenever any sign(s) associated with EPM are noticed. Horses which receive prompt, aggressive treatment early in the course of the disease have the best chance for complete recovery.

> **AT A GLANCE**
>
> - Keeping a horse physically and mentally healthy can help it resist infection.
> - Call your vet promptly when a horse exhibits any signs associated with EPM.
> - Limit the access of opossums to the horse's environment as much as possible.
> - Avoid travel stress by planning in advance, providing adequate hydration, and keeping all vaccinations current.
> - Studies of past and future cases of EPM should help determine which management practices and environmental factors contribute to the development of EPM.
> - Development of an EPM vaccine is a possibility at some point.

FACILITY MAINTENANCE

The condition and layout of physical facilities can help avoid injuries and reduce exposure to EPM. Horse-friendly design and construction and routine maintenance will help prevent physical stress due to injury and bacterial infection that can predispose horses to EPM.

It is important to limit the access of opossums in the horse's environment as much as possible. Individual opossums cover a fairly small territory during their lives (approximately one square mile). They are prolific and have an average lifespan of three years. They live much longer in captivity because it is much easier to avoid their No. 1 predator: the automobile. Because a single female can produce up to 30 offspring a year, local populations can become quite dense. Many assume that a local opossum problem does not exist because opossums are rarely seen on the property. However, they are nocturnal and are rarely seen alive during the day.

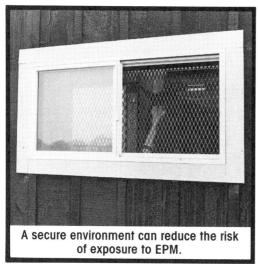

A secure environment can reduce the risk of exposure to EPM.

Opossums have a ravenous appetite and will eat virtually anything. It is important to keep the area clean. Pet food, garbage, and anything edible (dead birds and rodents) should be kept inaccessible. Livestock feeds, including hay and grain, should be stored away from opossums.

Unattractive wire fencing designed to prevent opossums from entering pastures is available. Live trapping and relocation of opossums should be attempted to reduce sporocyst contamination of the area. Horse feed should be kept clean and as free of bugs as possible. Extrusion and some pelleting processes produce sufficient heat to kill sporocysts present in the ingredients. It is not known if this represents a significant source of sporocyst exposure. Fly control might be helpful. Covering barn openings with hardware cloth, which is easier to maintain than screen, will prevent the entry of opossums and birds. Methods to limit fecal contamination of outdoor water sources from opossums and birds should be considered.

TRAVEL PLANNING

Long trailer rides are extremely stressful and are commonly mentioned in the clinical history of horses that develop EPM. Plans should be made in advance to avoid travel stress. Adequate hydration is essential.

Vaccinations should be up to date to avoid stress associated with various contagious diseases. It also is important to minimize corticosteroid use to avoid immune suppression. Many horses travel extensively and are dependent on the feed and water supplies at various local facilities. It is important to consider the potential for exposure under these circumstances and to plan ahead to avoid exposure at your destination.

RESEARCH IN PROGRESS: RISK FACTOR ANALYSIS AND VACCINES

Risk Factor Analysis

Ongoing and proposed retrospective (past EPM cases) and prospective (future EPM cases) studies at The Ohio State University and Michigan State University have been mentioned previously. These studies will help determine which management practices and environmental factors contribute to the development of clinical disease and promote appropriate control.

Vaccine development

The development of vaccines to protect against protozoal parasites is extremely difficult. However, significant progress has been made toward effective vaccine development against protozoal diseases of other animals. Recent advancements in our ability to test potential vaccines in the horse makes it possible to be optimistic for progress in this area. Several university research groups are searching actively for protective components of *S. neurona*. This work also might lead to effective immunotherapy, whether or not a vaccine becomes a reality in the next few years.

FREQUENTLY ASKED QUESTIONS

What is EPM?

Equine protozoal myeloencephalitis is the most commonly diagnosed neurologic disease of horses in North America. Clinical signs are caused by infection of the brain and spinal cord with the protozoal parasite *Sarcocystis neurona*.

How do horses get EPM?

Opossums shed infective *S. neurona* sporocysts in their feces. Horses become infected by ingesting sporocysts in contaminated food or water.

Is EPM contagious?

Sarcocystis infections are not contagious. Parasite survival requires alternating infection of a meat eater and its prey or carrion. The infective stage for the predator or scavenger only develops in the tissues of the appropriate prey or carrion. The life cycle of *S. neurona* cannot be completed in the horse. The infectious stage for the opossum does not develop. The horse is considered a dead-end host. The true intermediate host is believed to include a variety of birds, but this remains uncertain.

Why are only some horses affected?

A number of factors are believed to contribute to the development of clinical disease. These include the number of parasites ingested, the horse's immune status, and stress. Large parasite doses are required to induce experimental infections. It seems reasonable to assume that natural infections are similar. Immunity can be compromised by some medications, various diseases, and stress. Stress can result from heavy exercise, injury, long distance travel, pregnancy, or mental distress.

How can I tell if my horse has EPM?

The clinical signs of EPM are quite variable. However, the most common clinical signs include progressive incoordination of the rear limbs and weakness. A complete neurologic examination and laboratory testing are the most effective means of diagnosis.

What does a positive EPM test mean?

The EPM test detects antibodies that are specific for *S. neurona* in the blood or spinal fluid of horses. The presence of specific antibodies in blood indicates that the horse has been exposed to the parasite. However, exposure is quite common. The horse might never develop EPM. Horses with other neurologic diseases frequently test positive for exposure to *S. neurona*. A positive spinal fluid sample indicates that the parasite has entered the CNS unless the sample is blood contaminated. This is a strong indication that clinical signs are due to EPM.

Should EPM testing be done pre-purchase?

Not in my opinion. Exposure is too common. A positive blood test is of little concern.

Spinal fluid testing is not recommended for normal horses. Test results cannot be interpreted reliably.

Question & Answer

Can EPM be treated?

Effective treatment is available. It should be started quickly to provide maximum benefit.

Is treatment expensive?

Optimal treatment is relatively expensive. The cost of treatment includes diagnosis and management, as well as appropriate medication. Medication and supplements alone can cost $250-$1,000 a month, depending on the treatment regimen prescribed.

Can I continue to work my horse during treatment?

Every situation is unique. Severely affected horses should be confined to help prevent further injury. Horses with adequate mobility appear to benefit from light exercise. However, stress reduces the horse's ability to fight infection. In my opinion, heavy work or full training should be avoided while horses are on medication and continuing to show improvement.

Will my horse eventually recover?

It is impossible to predict on an individual basis. Mildly affected horses which are diagnosed quickly and receive prompt treatment have the best chance to make a full recovery. Severely affected horses and those that have had clinical signs for many weeks often show significant improvement, but are more likely to have some residual neurologic deficits. It has been estimated that up to 75% of treated horses show improvement and that less than 25% recover completely.

What can I do to prevent EPM?

The parasite is spread by opossums. Relocation of opossums away from horses and protection of feed and water from fecal contamination should help reduce the risk of exposure.

Should I treat my horse periodically to prevent disease?

It is not advisable. Short-term (less than 90 days) periodic treatment might result in the development of drug resistant parasite strains in your horse. If clinical disease does develop, it will be more difficult to treat.

Are researchers working on a cure or a vaccine for EPM?

Yes. Several groups are working on improved treatments and vaccine development. EPM can cause permanent CNS damage prior to diagnosis. Therefore, a cure is not really possible, only more effective medications. Vaccine development will be difficult. *Sarcocystis neurona* is much more complex genetically than a virus or bacteria. Although it is unlikely that a vaccine will ever be able to prevent infection completely, it might be possible to improve a horse's ability to eliminate the parasite before it causes clinical disease.

GLOSSARY

Antibody / Immunoglobulin — specialized proteins which are custom-made by white blood cells to help fight specific infectious agents.

Apicomplexa — a large grouping (Phylum) of intracellular protozoal parasites that each contains an apical complex for penetration into host cells

Ataxia — incoordinated movement

Atrophy — loss of muscle mass

Axon — a long, narrow process which extends from a neuron and transmits nerve impulses

Blood-brain barrier — tightly joined layer of cells lining central nervous system blood vessels which prevent blood components from entering the cerebrospinal fluid

Bradyzoite — slowly dividing asexual stage of *Sarcocystis* found in sarcocysts; infectious stage for the definitive host

Central nervous system — Brain, brainstem, and spinal cord

Cerebrospinal fluid — colorless fluid which acts like a "shock-absorber" to protect the central nervous system from injury

Cervical spine — that part of the spinal column from the base of the skull to the shoulders

Cranial nerves — set of 12 peripheral nerves originating from the brainstem that control sight, smell, taste, hearing, balance, chewing, swallowing, and muscles of the face, eyes, and shoulders.

Definitive host — the animal host that harbors the sexual stages of parasite reproduction

Differential diagnoses — a list of diseases most likely to be responsible for the clinical signs observed

Epidemiology — the study of disease in a population rather than an individual

Encephalitis — infection of the brain

Gray matter — concentrated area of neurons in the central nervous system which appear gray

Immune System — body defense network made up of several specialized white blood cell types which are spread throughout the body to recognize foreign invaders and attack them directly or by releasing specific antibodies

Immunoblot analysis — method used for the current EPM test which detects antibodies directed against parasite-specific proteins in the serum or CSF of infected horses

Incubation period — the length of time between parasite (sporocyst) ingestion and the onset of clinical signs

Inflammation — a non-specific process activated in response to infectious agents or injuries in an effort to eliminate the invader or repair of the injured area; characterized by swelling, redness, and pain outside CNS

Intermediate host — animal host that harbors the asexually dividing forms of *Sarcocystis* or other parasites

Motor neuron — nerve cell located in the central nervous system which sends nerve impulses that initiate muscle activity

Lumbar spine — portion of the spinal column in the small of the back.

Glossary

Merozoite — generic term referring to individual parasites produced by asexual multiplication (bradyzoites and tachyzoites are both merozoites)

Myelitis — infection of the spinal cord

Myeloencephalitis — infection of the spinal cord and brain

Myeloencephalopathy — non-infectious disease process of the spinal cord and brain

Neospora caninum — apicomplexan protozoa that causes equine abortion and might rarely infect the central nervous system

Neurologic examination — a thorough, systematic physical evaluation of the nervous system

PCR — polymerase chain reaction, a diagnostic and research technique designed to amplify very small amounts of DNA into easily detectable amounts

Peripheral nerve — all nerves outside the central nervous system

Proprioception — ability to sense limb position

Protozoa — very small, single-celled animals which can be parasitic

Risk factor — a circumstance which predisposes animals to exposure or the actual development of a disease

Sacrum — a single bone formed by the fusion of five to six vertebrae which attach the end of the spinal column to the pelvis

Sarcocyst — a large grouping (cyst) of bradyzoites located in the muscles of the intermediate host

Sarcocystis fayeri — species of *Sarcocystis* which cycles between horses and canines which may cause muscle soreness in horses

Sarcocystis neurona — the causative agent of EPM; the opossum is the definitive host; the intermediate host is uncertain

Sarcocystis falcatula — species of *Sarcocystis* which cycles between opossums and various birds

Sensory neuron — neurons located outside the central nervous system which send signals from the periphery back to the central nervous system

Seroprevalence — the percent of a population with antibodies to a particular infectious agent

Spinal nerve — nerves branching directly from the spinal cord to the rest of the body

Tachyzoite — rapidly dividing stage of *Sarcocystis* which develops in the walls of blood vessels of the intermediate host; stage of *S. neurona* responsible for causing EPM

Sporocyst — the stage of *Sarcocystis* produced in opossum intestines and shed into the environment to infect the intermediate host

Thoracic spine — that part of the spine from the shoulders to the small of the back

Vascular Endothelium — a layer of cells lining blood vessels throughout the body

White matter — central nervous system tissue made up almost entirely of axons

INDEX

Anti-inflammatory treatment 59

Ataxia..40

Atrophy...41

Bradyzoite 19

Cauda equina syndrome 60

Central nervous system.................19

Cerebrospinal fluid.......................62

Cervical vertebral
  myeloencephalopathy (CVM)..46

Clinical signs.................................41

Cranial nerves...............................37

Definitive host 21

Diagnosis.......................................37

Diclazuril 83

Differential diagnoses 46

Epidemiology................................23

EPM test...63

EPM test sensitivity/specificity 64

Equine degenerative myeloencephalopathy (EDM)................57

Equine herpesvirus myeloencephalopathy (EHV-1) 58

Exposure 27

Glossary...92

Immune response 26

Immunoblot analysis....................64

Incubation period.........................22

Inflammation.................................37

Intermediate host 17

Laboratory testing.........................62

Life cycle 13

Middle ear infection.....................58

Merozoite 13

Neoplasia.......................................61

Neospora caninum......................65

Neurologic examination 44

96

Opossum 11	*Sarcocystis neurona* 8
Otitis Media 58	*Sarcocystis falcatula* 19
PCR 68	Seroprevalence 27
Polyneuritis equi 60	Sporocyst 11
Prevention 84	Sulfa drugs 76
Protozoa 12	Tachyzoite 18
Pyrimethamine 76	Trauma 48
Rabies 60	Treatment 77
Relapse 77	Trimethoprim 76
Risk factors 23	Tumor 61
Sarcocyst 18	Verminous encephalomyelitis 59
Sarcocystis 13	Vitamin E 81
Sarcocystis fayeri 13	Wobbler 46

RECOMMENDED READINGS

Andrews, FM, Granstrom, DE, Provenza, M. Differentiation of neurological diseases in the horse by the use of albumin quotient and IgG index determination. Proceedings American Association of Equine Practitioners, Lexington, Ky. 1995; 41:215-217.

Bentz BG, Granstrom DE, Stamper S. Seroprevalence of antibodies to *Sarcocystis neurona* in horses residing in a county of southeastern Pennsylvania. Journal American Veterinary Medical Association. 1996; 210:517-518.

Blythe LL, Granstrom DE, Hansen DE, Walker LL, Bartlett J, Stamper S. Seroprevalence of antibodies to *Sarcocystis neurona* in horses residing in Oregon. Journal American Veterinary Medical Association. 1997; 210:525-527.

Fenger CK, Granstrom DE, Gajadhar, et al. Experimental induction of equine protozoal myeloencephalitis in horses using *Sarcocystis* sp. Sporocysts from the opossum (*Didelphis virginiana*). Veterinary Parasitology. 1997; 68:199-217.

Fenger CK, Granstrom DE, Langemeier JL, et al. Identification of Opossums (*Didelphis virginiana*) as the putative definitive host of *Sarcocystis neurona*. Journal of Parasitology. 1995; 81:916-919.

Fenger, CK. "Treating Equine Protozoal Myelitis." The Horse: Your Guide To Equine Health Care. June, 1995;18-20.

Granstrom DE, Dubey JP, Giles RC, et al. Equine protozoal myeloencephalitis: Biology and epidemiology. In: Nakajima H, Plowright W, eds. Proceedings VII International Conference of Equine Infectious Diseases. Tokyo, Japan: R & W Publications Ltd., Newmarket, UK. 1994:109-111.

Granstrom DE, Reed SM. Equine Protozoal Myeloencephalitis. Equine Practice. 1994; 16:23-26.

Granstrom DE. Equine protozoal myeloencephalitis: Review of 1993 and 1994. Proceedings American Association of Equine Practitioners. Lexington, Ky. 1995:218-219.

Granstrom, DE. "EPM Seminar." The Horse: Your Guide To Equine Health Care. November, 1995:14-23.

Granstrom DE. Recent advances in the laboratory diagnosis of equine parastici diseases. Veterinary Clinics of North America. 1995; 11:437-442.

Granstrom DE. Equine protozoal myeloencephalitis. Veterinary Forum. 1996; 7:52-57.

Granstrom DE, Saville, WJ. Equine protozoal myeloencephalitis. In: Equine Internal Medicine, SM Reed and WM Bayley Eds., WB Saunders, Co. Philadelphia, Penn., in press.

Grayson Foundation Stages EPM Conference. Grayson-Jockey Club Research Foundation, Inc.; 1996.

Herbert, KS. "EPM." The Horse: Your Guide To Equine Health Care. March, 1995:24-27.

Herbert, KS. "EPM: Hope At Last." The Horse: Your Guide To Equine Health Care. April, 1997:47-54.

Herbert, KS and Becht, J, DVM, Diplomate ACVIM. "Dealing With EPM Horses: One Veterinarian's Experience." The Horse: Your Guide To Equine Health Care. September, 1995:24-28.

Moore B, Granstrom DE, Reed S. Diagnosis of equine protozoal myeloencephalitis and cervical stenotic myelopathy. Compendium of Continuing Education for Practicing Veterinarians. 1995: 17:419-426.

Reed SM, Granstrom D, Rivas LJ, Saville WA, Moore BR, Mitten LA. Results of cerebrospinal fluid analysis in 119 horses testing positive to the Western blot test on both serum and CSF to equine protozoal encephalomyelitis. Proceedings American Association of Equine Practitioners. Vancouver, BC; 1994:199.

Reed, SM, Kohn CW, Hinchcliff KW, et al. Clinical findings and cerebrospinal fluid analysis including Western blot analysis on horses presented for neurologic disease at The Ohio State University. In: DeNovo R, ed. Proceedings American College of Veterinary Internal Medicine Forum. 13 ed. Lake Buena Vista, Fla. 1995:739-741.

Reed SM, Saville WJA. Equine Protozoal Encephalomyelitis. In: Zinninger SE ed. Proceedings American Association of Equine Practitioners. Denver, Colo. 1996:75-79.

Saville WJ, Reed SM, Granstrom DE, Hinchcliff KW, Kohn CW, Stamper S. Abstract: Prevalence of serum antibodies to *Sarcocystis neurona* in horses in Ohio. Proceedings American Association of Equine Practitioners. Lexington, Ky; 1995:220-221.

EPM sites on the Internet

- Equine Protozoal Myeloencephalitis (EPM) Research at
  The Ohio State University
  http://prevmed.vet.ohio-state.edu/epm/index.htm
- Equine Protozoal Myeloencephalitis (EPM) from
  The University of Kentucky Equine Parasitology

http://www.uky.edu/Agriculture/VetScience/Parasitology/epmhome.htm

Articles on the Internet

- http://www.uky.edu/Agriculture/VetScience/Parasitology/publst.htm
- http://www.thehorse.com/current/epm0497.html
- http://www.freerein.com/epm/epm.html

Picture Credits

INTRODUCTION
Dr. David E. Granstrom, 12, 14.

CHAPTER ONE
Dr. Neil M. Williams, 18; Dr. David E. Granstrom, 19; Barbara D. Livingston, 25; Anne M. Eberhardt, 26; *The Blood-Horse*, 30; Dr. Zhao Xiaomin, 31.

CHAPTER TWO
Dr. David E. Granstrom, 38; Anne M. Eberhardt, 39; Cheryl Manista, 40.

CHAPTER THREE
Anne M. Eberhardt, 49, 50, 51, 55, 62, 67; Dr. Josie Traub, 49; Dr. Neil M. Williams, 49; Hagyard-Davidson-McGee, 51; Dr. David E. Granstrom, 52, 53, 56; Cheryl Manista, 54, 55; Dr. Mary Rose Paradis, 55.

CHAPTER FOUR
Anne M. Eberhardt, 80, 82; Equipix, 81; Cheryl Manista, 83.

CHAPTER FIVE
Anne M. Eberhardt, 84; *The Blood-Horse*, 86.

COVER/BOOK DESIGN — SUZANNE C. DEPP
ILLUSTRATIONS — ROBIN PETERSON
COVER PHOTOGRAPH — CHERYL MANISTA

About the Author

David E. Granstrom, DVM, PhD, is considered the foremost authority on the subject of equine protozoal myeloencephalitis (EPM). While at the University of Kentucky, Granstrom developed the first test able to detect the presence of the parasite that causes EPM and oversaw further advancements in the diagnosis of the disease. He has written book chapters on EPM, and his articles on the subject have appeared in numerous veterinary journals.

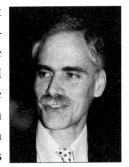
David E. Granstrom

Granstrom has a degree in veterinary medicine and a PhD in parasitology from Kansas State University. He began his career in 1978 with a private veterinary practice in Laurie, Missouri, taught at Kansas State, then joined the University of Kentucky in 1988, first as an assistant then an associate professor. Since May of 1997, Granstrom has been assistant director of education and research for the American Veterinary Medical Association. He and his family live in suburban Chicago.